making aromatherapy
creams &
lotions

101 Natural
Formulas to
Revitalize &
Nourish Your Skin

Donna Maria

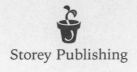

Storey Publishing

*The mission of Storey Publishing is to serve our customers by
publishing practical information that encourages
personal independence in harmony with the environment.*

Edited by Deborah Balmuth and Robin Catalano
Cover design by Betty Kodela
Cover photograph by © Nick Klements / FPG
Text design and production by Jennifer Jepson Smith
Photographs by Giles Prett, except on pages 2, 14, 27, 28, 34, 44, 54, 56, 57, 59,
   66, 85, 91, 94, 104, 106, 121, 126, 127, and 139 © PhotoDisk, Inc.; pages 5,
   22, 62, 88, 102, and 107 © Joe Atlas for Artville; pages 11, 64, 70, 79, 82, and
   92 © Eyewire Images; pages iii, 36, 38, 41, 109, 112, 130, 132, 140, 150 © Jeff
   Burke and Lorraine Triolo for Artville; pages 20 and 31 © Quarto, Inc. for Artville
Photo imaging by Erin Lincourt
Indexed by Nina Forrest, Looking Up Indexing Service

The information in this book is true and complete to the best of our knowledge. All recommendations are made without guarantee on the part of the author or Storey Publishing.
The author and publisher disclaim any liability in connection with the use of this information. For additional information, please contact Storey Publishing, 210 MASS MoCA Way,
North Adams, MA 01247.

Storey books are available for special premium and promotional uses and for customized
editions. For further information, please call (800) 793-9396.

Printed in the United States by Versa Press
20 19 18 17 16 15 14 13 12 11

Library of Congress Cataloging-in-Publication Data

Coles Johnson, Donna Maria, 1962–
     Making aromatherapy creams and lotions : 101 natural formulas to
     revitalize and nourish your skin / Donna Maria Coles Johnson.
                          p.   cm.
     ISBN 978-1-58017-241-7 (pbk. : alk. paper)
     1. Skin—Care and hygiene. 2. Herbal cosmetics. 3. Aromatherapy.
     I. Title.
RL87 .C65 2000
615'.321—dc21   00-023881
                                                                        CIP

Contents

Dedication

I humbly acknowledge my Lord and Savior, Jesus the Christ.
This book is dedicated to my Forever Friend,
Robin Maryl Greene Peel Turner.

~

Acknowledgments

Thanks to my precious husband, Darryl, whose unconditional love and unfailing friendship bring me great joy.

Mom, Daddy, Jeffrey, and Christopher: As your daughter and sister, I am grateful for your constant presence and love.

Nan, my Aromatic Mother, who shares with me everything she learns about life, and who introduced me to the world of aromatherapy. Aura, whose faith and wisdom constantly remind me that "this is not about me." Terri, my voice of reason when my pity parties get out of hand. Sabrina, who brings perspective and acceptance into my life.

Nancy Welch and Jennifer Betts, whose recipe testing and filling in for a broken computer will always be remembered. My editors, Deborah Balmuth and Robin Catalano, whose professionalism and patience have made it possible for me to speak to people around the world. Paige Eversole McMahon of McMahon Communications, whose ingenuity and communication skills are beyond compare.

Caroline Mulligan, Karen Samara, and Tanya Fleck, who supported me when I opened Maria Grace Aromatherapy Shop in 1993. Lisa Smith, who willingly smears everything I make all over her face and is a most valued friend. To Ingrid Poplett, Vicki Kgasoane, and the women of South Africa's Alexandra Township, sharing with you was a great privilege. You are a fragrant aroma of the beauty of your native land. To the Aromatic Beauty Workshop participants, thank you for allowing me to share with you the earth's fragrant bounty. To the members of the Handmade Toiletries Network, thanks for partnering with me to secure the future of the handmade toiletries industry.

And to my aromatic mentors, who have inspired and encouraged me, and who have generously shared their experiences: Pamela Parsons, Rachael Shapiro, Jade Shutes, Gabriel Mojay, Kurt Schnaubelt, Anastasia Crabtree, Ricey Clapp, Leslie Plant, and Jan Salko. And thanks to Eugenia, wherever you are.

Preface: The Birth of a Cosmeti-Cook

When I was a little girl, Sunday evenings at home were very exciting. After one of my mother's awesome dinners, Daddy typically announced that he was going to the neighborhood pharmacy. This simple declaration left me brimming with anticipation, for it meant that while he purchased household necessities, I could happily meander through the Supreme Pharmacy Aisle (SPA for short), where aromatic creams, soaps, lotions, and potions of all kinds were displayed from floor to ceiling.

Daddy always seemed both pleased and amused to purchase a fragrant lotion or cream for me. I could hardly wait to get home so I could use the goodies in one sitting while my parents watched *Sixty Minutes* and *The Flip Wilson Show*.

Few experiences since have compared to the preadolescent delight I enjoyed when I used my own money to purchase a sweet-smelling cosmetic called Green Apple Peel-Off Facial Mask. It was appropriately light green in color and contained little shimmering "moisture pearls" to soothe and nourish my skin. The smell was to die for.

While the mask dried on my skin, I closed my eyes and fancied myself a world-famous model with a flawless complexion and perfectly conditioned hair.

My interest in toiletries grew tremendously in college, when I learned that the concoctions I had kneaded into my skin for years contained all sorts of things that were anything but good for me. One day at a library, I stumbled across a book on making natural cosmetics. From that moment on, inspired by shapes, people, odors, music, dance, textures, and colors, I have been inexplicably led from one aromatic cocktail to another in an endlessly pleasant cycle of fragrant creation and renewal. Whether it's lotion or soap, foaming gel or lip balm, flowers suspended in oil or body cream the color of pink cotton candy and pistachio ice cream — if it rubs, rolls, smooths, or spritzes on, I want to try it.

This book is born of a desire to share my aromatic experiences (and those of other people), to encourage and inspire you to craft quality natural skin-care products for home use that rival those found at the most exclusive department stores and salons, and to incorporate in the recipes some of the world's rarest aromatic oils. I hope you enjoy making them as much as I have enjoyed creating them.

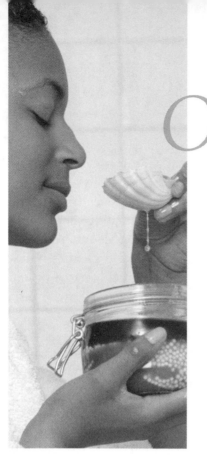

One:

Aromatic Self-Care

*I*nterest in the use of natural aromatic oils has risen steadily over the past quarter-century as people have grown increasingly weary of the traditional treatments for ailments from minor skin problems to chronic fatigue and depression. Homeopathy, reflexology, herbalism, flower essence therapy, iridology, acupuncture, massage therapy, and many other complementary forms of alternative care are now available. If used responsibly, these modalities allow us to play a more active role in maintaining our health and well-being.

A significant outgrowth of the renewed interest in nonconventional self-care is the fascinating rediscovery of a cousin to the centuries-old practice of using aromatic oils to positively affect the human condition. Today, this practice is typically called *aromatherapy,* and its proper definition and scope are the subjects of considerable international discussion and debate. The most widely accepted description of aromatherapy encompasses the blending of plant essential oils to promote health, beauty, and well-being. This book concentrates on the incorporation of essential oils in combination with other natural plant extracts, both aromatic and unscented, into handmade skin-care products.

What Are Aromatic Oils?

Aromatic oils are removed by various extraction techniques from leaves, petals, blossoms, barks, twigs, and other fragrant plant parts. Different extraction techniques produce diverse types of oils with different chemical makeups and uses. For example, rose essential oil extracted via the steam distillation method is very different from rose absolute, which is extracted with solvents. These differences do not necessarily mean that one oil is superior to another, but they often indicate the suitability of the oil for a particular purpose.

There are several types of aromatic oils, including essential oils and absolutes. Essential oils have historically been considered the purest form of aromatic plant material because they are extracted without solvents. As such, they are the oils most frequently used for skin-care purposes, and the most readily available. For the sake of ease, I typically use the term *aromatic oils* to refer to aromatic oils collectively and am more specific about types of oils as necessary.

I bent down to the vine, shaking to drink in its honey
and its flower and my thoughts like heavy grapes,
bramble-thick my breath — I could not,
as I breathed, choose among the scents, but culled them all,
and drank them as one drinks joy or sorrow
suddenly sent by fate. I drank them all.

— Angelos Silcelianus, *The First Rain*

Jan Berger, Body Way
Boulder, Colorado

For Jan, making a cream for a friend is more than just combining proper ingredients and amounts. Rather, it is a loving expression of tender feelings that, in combination with the gentle plant oils she uses, serves to encourage and uplift the user. Jan's creation of a product she calls Vicki's Voice illustrates this point.

Vicki often experienced extreme anger and frustration and spent much of her time "screaming" inside. She expressed her anguish to Jan, who created a cream that combines essential oils with other plant materials. When Vicki applies the cream, she is reminded of the care taken to create it just for her. She remembers that she has freedom of voice and is able to express her feelings, whatever they are, and to make conscious decisions to laugh, speak, scream, or cry. This freedom allows Vicki to live a life in which her feelings no longer shackle her but are legitimate expressions of her individuality and humanity.

Until Jan started making lotions and creams, she hated spending time in the kitchen, which she described as the coldest place in her childhood home. Today, the formerly laborious chores of measuring, calculating ingredient amounts, and stirring are a stimulating part of the creative process. Jan's Boulder kitchen, where she concocts fabulous formulas for her company, Body Way, is her aromatic playpen.

My favorite Body Way product is Petal Play, a cream with the look and feel of white chocolate mousse.

Taking the All-Natural Approach

The benefits of incorporating aromatic oils and other unadulterated plant extracts into handmade toiletries are as diverse as the hundreds of plants from which the aromatics are taken, and can vary greatly from person to person. Some people experience the greatest satisfaction when they find the perfect blend of aromas to suit their taste or mood, while others enjoy the process of creating the base product regardless of the final aroma. Still others are most concerned about the effects of the aromatic oils on their skin and will sacrifice a pleasant smell to obtain the desired therapeutic effect. In any case, using aromatic ingredients from faraway lands to create potions that nourish both body and soul continues to be a time-honored and universal pleasure.

The recipes in this book call for pure and genuine aromatic plant oils, which I highly recommend to achieve maximum skin-care benefits. Though some people will no doubt be allergic to or otherwise adversely affected by certain pure oils, the likelihood of irritation is significantly reduced with these oils in comparison to synthetic oils. In addition, since you choose the ingredients, you can remove the offending ingredient(s) by a careful process of trial and error.

Some pure aromatic oils can be pricey, and synthetic fragrance oils can be used. Bear in mind, however, that the possibility of an adverse skin reaction is also increased if synthetic ingredients are used.

Blending and Using Essential Oils

When making handmade skin-care products, you can combine different aromatic oils to create products designed to address very specific skin conditions. In addition, because many aromatic oils are used to affect mood and health, you can select different oils on the basis of your state of health and mind. A classic example is lavender essential oil, which is not only an excellent skin conditioner but also a gentle relaxant.

One of the distinguishing characteristics of an aromatic oil is its volatility rate, which affects not only how long its aroma lasts but also how its odor changes as it is exposed to air. Thus, a combination of three oils that are each known to quickly vaporize will be simplistic and short-lived. On the other hand, a combination of three oils with varying volatility rates will produce a mellifluous fragrance that beautifully highlights the individual characteristics of each oil.

The differences in oil volatility rates form the basis of the art of perfumery. So if your goal is to design a skin-care product to suit a particular skin type, and you also wish to take into account the fragrance of the finished product, you will want to consider the volatility rates of the oils you use. This is most often described by the particular "note" category into which the oil falls. These notes can be likened to the instruments in a symphony orchestra.

Top notes are the flutes and wind chimes of an aromatic blend and are composed chiefly of citrus oils. They are light and sweet, and the first inhalation immediately reveals their delicate and playful nature. Top notes can be sharp and haughty, and they always tend toward extremely high levels of volatility and mischievous activity. They vaporize quickly, though they continue to tease us with their playfulness by peeking out now and again.

Middle notes are the clarinets and violins of the aromatic symphony. They are the character of the blend, if you will, providing support for the top notes and lift and clarity for the base notes.

Base or bottom notes are the basses, bassoons, and timpani of the combination. They are mysterious, heavy, deep, and strong, with an extremely low volatility rate. Base notes are typically imperceptible at first, but without them, the top and middle notes would battle it out until they both simply dissolved into the air.

Sometimes an oil can take on different characteristics because of the other oils in the blend. For instance, lavender makes a wonderful middle note when combined with several citrus oils and fewer base notes. On the other hand, lavender oil performs more like a top note when mixed with several base notes and fewer top notes.

Command Performance: Aromatics in Concert

Depending on the oils they are combined with, many aromatic oils can belong to more than one section of the orchestra. Use the classifications provided here as guidelines for creating your own aromatic blends. All ingredients are essential oils unless otherwise noted, and oils not typically used in the making of perfume have been excluded.

TOP NOTES

Bergamot, grapefruit, lemon, mandarin, melissa, orange

TOP/MIDDLE NOTES

Carrot seed, Roman and German chamomile, clary sage, geranium, helichrysum, lavender, myrtle, neroli, palmarosa, rose, rose geranium, rosemary, zdravetz

MIDDLE/BASE NOTES

Beeswax absolute, calendula CO_2, carnation absolute, cypress, jasmine absolute, mimosa absolute, rose absolute and concrete, rose hips CO_2, rosewood, sea buckthorn berry CO_2, spikenard, tuberose absolute, violet leaf CO_2, ylang ylang, zdravetz

BASE NOTES

Frankincense, jasmine absolute, myrrh, oakmoss, oakmoss absolute, patchouli, sandalwood, vanilla absolute, vetiver

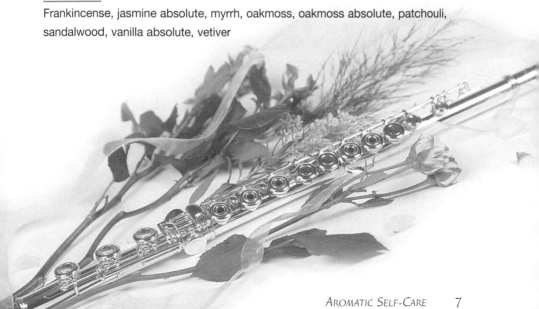

Safety Precautions for Aromatic Oils

When used properly, aromatic plant oils are healing on a variety of levels. Although natural, these oils are extremely concentrated and must be used with caution. Take the time to become acquainted with their individual properties, cautions, and recommended uses.

Bear in mind that the guidelines for using aromatic plant oils are constantly evolving as additional research is conducted. In general, I offer these basic recommendations:

- Because the quality and purity of aromatic oils range from superb to abysmal, as a rule I do not recommend ingestion of aromatic oils. Use these oils internally only upon the specific recommendation of a qualified aromatherapist.
- Do not allow aromatic oils to come into direct contact with your eyes or other mucous membranes. Use oils on broken or irritated skin only after consultation with a qualified aromatherapist or your health-care practitioner.
- Always conduct a patch test before using any beauty product to ensure that you are not sensitive or allergic to particular ingredients. See page 58 for instructions.
- Do not use aromatic oils undiluted on the skin unless recommended by a qualified aromatherapist — with the exceptions of very small amounts of lavender and tea tree essential oils.
- If you are pregnant, wish to become pregnant, are under the continuous care of a health-care provider, or take any medications, it is wise to seek medical advice before using particular aromatic oils. Be aware of your body's changing needs, and act accordingly.
- If you encounter any adverse reactions after using aromatic oils for any purpose, seek the advice of a qualified health-care provider, a trained aromatherapist, or even emergency medical personnel immediately.

Creating Aromatic Alchemy

Bearing in mind that no one formula suits everyone, I have created seven different Aromatic Alchemy blends for you to add to the skin-care products you make using the formulas in this book.

To make the blends, first use separate droppers to measure each aromatic oil. Place the drops of oil into a clean glass bottle, and shake gently to mix. Allow the blend to sit for a few days to "mellow" before use.

Aroma News

Here are some interesting facts about fragrance:
- *Some shopping malls pipe bakery smells, believed to trigger the buying impulse, through their ventilation systems.*
- *Because of the chemicals used in commercial perfumes, a few municipalities in Canada have enacted scent-free zoning regulations prohibiting people from wearing perfume in public places.*
- *Casinos often use relaxing aromas to encourage gamblers to linger longer and gamble more.*
- *Some Paris Métro stops are perfumed with Madeleine, a citrus, floral, and musk aroma.*
- *Shiseido, a Japanese cosmetics firm, recently introduced a fragrance specifically designed to mask what the Japanese often describe as the peculiar body odor of aging men.*
- *The smell of freshly mowed grass is piped into some of the terminals at London's Heathrow Airport.*

THE CO$_2$ CREW

Each of the blends in this chapter contains the CO$_2$ Crew. The CO$_2$ Crew adds remarkable anti-inflammatory, rejuvenating, and healing qualities to each Aromatic Alchemy blend. Depending on the other ingredients in the formula, it could also add a light golden tint. The CO$_2$ Crew finds its way into nearly everything I make.

1 part sea buckthorn berry CO$_2$ extract
1 part rose hips seed CO$_2$ select extract
1 part calendula CO$_2$ select extract

FACE FLOWERS

Use this blend for dry skin.
makes ⅛ ounce (3.5 g)

85 drops CO$_2$ Crew
30 drops German chamomile essential oil
25 drops rose essential oil
15 drops neroli essential oil
15 drops helichrysum essential oil
15 drops yarrow essential oil

A nose in a million. Over the years, with the proper training, this can be developed until it is capable of identifying even the ghost of a fragrance — the crucial drop that lifts a perfume from the ordinary to the unforgettable. But first, you have to find those talented nostrils.

— Peter Mayle, *Encore Provence*

Tender Warrior

This special blend can be used for any skin type.

makes ⅛ ounce (3.5 g)

50 drops geranium essential oil
40 drops CO_2 Crew
30 drops myrtle essential oil
30 drops lavender essential oil
20 drops sandalwood essential oil
25 drops rosemary (verbenone type) essential oil

Mercy

This blend helps soothe and heal cracked or inflamed skin.

makes ⅛ ounce (3.5 g)

100 drops CO_2 Crew
30 drops German chamomile essential oil
25 drops helichrysum essential oil
10 drops spikenard essential oil
10 drops patchouli essential oil

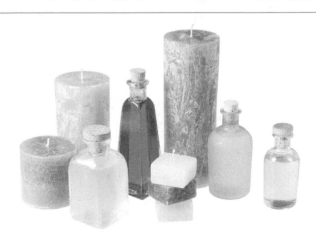

TONE THYME

Ideal for greasy, oily, or acne-prone skin.
makes ⅛ ounce (3.5 g)

50 drops lavender essential oil
30 drops geranium essential oil
25 drops CO_2 Crew
25 drops cypress essential oil
25 drops rosemary (verbenon type) essential oil
20 drops thyme (linalol type) essential oil
15 drops sandalwood essential oil
6 drops lemon essential oil
6 drops tea tree essential oil

BALANCING ACT

Add this to products designed for normal to oily skin.
makes ⅛ ounce (3.5 g)

50 drops lavender essential oil
30 drops CO_2 Crew
25 drops geranium essential oil
20 drops myrtle essential oil
15 drops tea tree essential oil
15 drops cypress essential oil
15 drops thyme (linalol type) essential oil
6 drops sandalwood essential oil
5 drops ylang ylang essential oil

DRENCH

This is an excellent blend for dry and/or mature skin.

makes ⅛ ounce (3.5 g)

70 drops CO_2 Crew
25 drops sandalwood essential oil
20 drops frankincense essential oil
25 drops myrrh essential oil
15 drops carrot seed essential oil
10 drops yarrow essential oil
5 drops rose essential oil
5 drops patchouli essential oil

SAVING FACE

Try this blend to boost the quality of sallow, lifeless skin.

makes ⅛ ounce (3.5 g)

75 drops CO_2 Crew
30 drops frankincense essential oil
25 drops lavender essential oil
25 drops myrrh essential oil
25 drops geranium essential oil
6 drops melissa essential oil

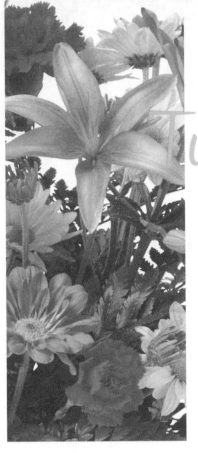

Two: The Aromatic Pantry

Your Aromatic Pantry should be stocked with ingredients that make your heart (and your skin) sing. Nature has ensured that there is no shortage of oils from which to choose, and one of the greatest blessings of life is this range of fragrant natural selections.

How Essential Oils Are Made

A variety of methods are employed to extract aromatic oils from plant materials. Among the most widely known are distillation and hydrodiffusion, mechanical expression, enfleurage, solvent extraction, and carbon dioxide (CO_2) extraction. Use the information given here to decide which type of aromatic oil best suits your purposes.

Steam Distillation and Hydrodiffusion

The most common method of extracting essential oils from plant material is steam distillation. The plant material is placed on a grate, which is then placed on top of (or into) boiling water in a large vat. The steam from the boiling water is forced through the plant material, causing it to rupture and release its aromatic constituents in vaporized form. The vapors rise and are passed through a condenser or set of cooling tanks, where they convert into liquid form. At the end of the distillation process, there are three distinct products:

- Spent plant material (discarded or used as compost)
- Essential oil
- Plant water, also called *hydrosol* or *hydrolat* (see page 61 for more information)

Although essential oils are purely natural extracts, the heat employed in the distillation process can destroy components that are present in the natural plant material. The distillation method can also produce some chemical constituents that are not present in the plant material in its natural state. For example, azulene, a valuable skin-soothing agent, is present in distilled German chamomile essential oil, but not in chamomile flowers.

Hydrodiffusion is far less common than steam distillation. In this process, steam is forced through the plant material from above rather than from underneath. Because this method tends to produce more water than does steam distillation, it is most useful when the desired output is plant water rather than plant oil.

Mechanical Expression

Mechanical expression extracts oils from the peel of citrus fruits. The process can be as simple as pressing on the plant with bare hands or as complex as placing the plant material in a large, porous drum that rotates rapidly enough to literally wrench out the aromatic oil. Though the expression process generates its own heat, the fact that no external heat source is used means that the oil produced has an aroma that is very true to the plant itself.

Enfleurage

Enfleurage is used to obtain aromatic oil from flower petals that cannot endure the heat of the distillation process. This process is rarely used today because it is expensive and labor-intensive.

Enfleurage involves the placement of individual flower petals on glass plates that have been smeared with a fatty substance, often a mixture of lard, suet, and benzoin (a preservative). After 24 to 48 hours, during which time the fat absorbs the aromatic oils from the flowers, the spent petals are replaced with fresh ones. The aromatic fat is then mixed with a solvent. The aromatic oil dissolves fully into the solvent, and the substance is filtered several times to remove the fat, which is discarded. Alcohol is then used to remove the solvent material, leaving behind an absolute, or fragrant oil.

Solvent Extraction: Absolutes, Concretes & Waxes

Absolutes and concretes are extracted via one of a number of petro-chemical solvents. These solvents have a lower boiling point than water and are most often used to extract aromatic oils from plant materials — often flower petals — that are too delicate to withstand the heat needed to distill essential oils. The plant material is placed on grills, which are lowered into the solvent material. As the solvent is heated, the flower oils, waxes, and color are dissolved into it. Once the spent flowers are removed, the aromatic slush is gently heated to evaporate the solvent. Further treatment using alcohol removes more of the solvent, and the remaining substance is called a concrete.

Concretes, which are often cold-stored until needed to produce an absolute, are further treated with solvents to separate out the aromatic oil and much of its color. When the extracted liquid, or absolute, is removed from the con-crete, primarily wax remains.

Wax can be used as a fragrant, effective thickener and binding agent in your

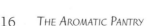

creams and lotions. However, because wax has limited commercial value, it has not always been treated to remove the residual solvent materials. Take special care when opening a new package, since any residual solvents can cause a light burning sensation in the lungs and nostrils.

There is great debate about the proper place of absolutes and concretes in both the aromatherapy and cosmetics industries. Consult reference books for further information regarding this ongoing professional discourse.

Carbon Dioxide Extraction

Carbon dioxide extraction removes aromatic oils without heat, instead applying very low pressure to the plant materials. The CO_2 extraction method produces oils that are reputed to retain most of the qualities of the whole plant, including fragrance, color, and chemical composition.

There are two distinct types of aromatic CO_2 oils:

Total CO_2 extracts are typically thick, tarlike substances that contain the plant's oils, along with waxes, fats, resins, and color. Bottles of total CO_2 extracts often must be held under warm water in order to achieve a pourable consistency. (I sometimes use a clean wooden stir stick or toothpick to remove total CO_2 extracts from their bottles.)

Select CO_2 extracts contain far less solid plant material, and their consistency, while still thick, is more like that of molasses. Select CO_2 extracts are a bit more expensive than total CO_2 extracts, in part because more of the plant material is discarded after completion of the select extraction process. I prefer these extracts; their consistency often makes them much easier to use.

Be sure to ask which type of CO_2 extract you are purchasing. If the supplier doesn't know, he should offer to find out. Purchase only from a supplier who can obtain this information for you. My favorite CO_2 extracts for skin care are rose hips seed, sea buckthorn berry, and calendula.

Solvent Extraction: Florasols

Florasols (formerly called *phytols* or *phytosols*) are produced using a fairly new extraction technique developed in the United Kingdom. Solvent extraction employs low-temperature tetrafluoroethane gas, a hydrofluorocarbon that is carefully and fully removed after the extraction process is complete.

The name *florasol* does not adequately describe the full range of oils that are available, including oils from nonfloral plant materials, such as cinnamon bark, bay leaf, orange peel, and nutmeg. Florasols are thought to be more concentrated than most other aromatic oils, capturing far more individual chemical components of the plant than other extraction methods. Perhaps this is the reason that, in my experience, much less florasol than essential oil and/or absolute is needed to scent a jar of cream.

Selecting and Storing Essential Oils

The ability to discern quality essential oils is developed over time; it cannot be effectively taught in a book. But an indispensable part of using essential oils safely and effectively is taking the time to learn about them, one or two at a time. In this way, you will begin to "know" the oils as you would a friend and will slowly learn to maximize their potential.

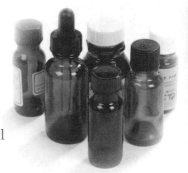

Purchasing Superior-Quality Oils

Among the chief frustrations expressed by my workshop participants are how difficult it is to know what to look for in a supplier of oils, how to recognize an inferior-quality oil, and what to do when suspicion arises about the purity of an oil. There is no substitute, especially for beginners, for ordering and comparing small quantities of the same oils from well-known suppliers. Admittedly, the learning curve is steep, and aromatherapy is not always an inexpensive venture. In my experience, however, quality does not always mean extreme expense. You must take the time to seek out quality oils that suit your needs and finances. If you begin with a few basic oils (many of which are used in the recipes in this book) and decide to enjoy the learning experience rather than expect to know everything by next week, you will soon be an "expert" in the oils you choose for your personal use. (See Resources for a list of suppliers that combine high-quality products with reasonable prices.)

Without a chemical analysis, there is no surefire way to determine the purity or components of a product labeled an essential oil. You could have an independent lab conduct an analysis, but the prices start at around $150 for one test. The good news is that as you work with essential oils, you will slowly be training your senses, especially your sense of smell, to distinguish exceptional oils. In addition, there are several questions you can ask to maximize your chances of purchasing high-quality oils. But first, you must take the time and accept the responsibility for educating yourself. The best place to start is a book on essential oils; check your local library or bookstore for titles. The Internet is also a good place to find information. Though neither medium is *always* reliable, they are excellent places to begin gathering information as you start your aromatic journey. If you are a beginner, I highly recommend that you start with *Aromatherapy: A Complete Guide to the Healing Art,* by Kathi Keville and Mindy Green.

Guidelines for Distinguishing Quality Oils

Once you have a basic arsenal of information, purchase about ½ ounce of two or three oils from two or three different suppliers. (*Note:* It is generally discourteous to use a supplier's toll-free order line to discuss the oils. Instead, call customer service and ask the supplier to set aside mutually convenient time for you to ask pertinent questions.) For your first purchase, I recommend lavender; eucalyptus; and a citrus oil, such as sweet orange or lemon. Each of these oils is versatile and has a pleasant aroma. Be sure that a single type of oil purchased from different suppliers comes from the same species of plant.

Here is a list of questions to use as a guideline in making essential oil purchases. You do not have to ask all of these questions; choose a few that are important to you and begin with those.

1. Are the oils pure, unadulterated extracts (also known as "genuine and authentic") from high-quality plant material? Oils that have been stretched with vegetable oils or other contaminants will not produce superb results in your skin-care products.

2. Where does the oil come from, and how was it extracted? Is the oil taken from organically grown plant material or from plants that were harvested in the wild? Knowing the method of extraction and country of origin can provide an idea of an oil's general aromatic characteristics and chemical makeup, each of which is influenced by climatic growing conditions, seasonal harvesting considerations, and other variables.

3. What part of the plant was the oil taken from? Juniper berry and clove bud oils are very different from their counterparts, juniper needle and clove leaf oils.

4. How does the supplier store oils? Storage habits are significant, since it is highly unlikely that your oil will be shipped to you immediately after it is received by the supplier. It is best to purchase oils that have been stored in dark-colored glass bottles, away from heat and sunlight, and that are as fresh as possible (unless you are after vintage frankincense!).

5. Is each oil individually priced on the basis of quantity purchased, harvesting technique, and other factors? Typically, the more oil you buy, the less you pay per ounce. Also, organically grown wildcrafted oils, which are generally preferred for maximum medicinal benefit, are usually more expensive than oils taken from plants grown using traditional farming methods.

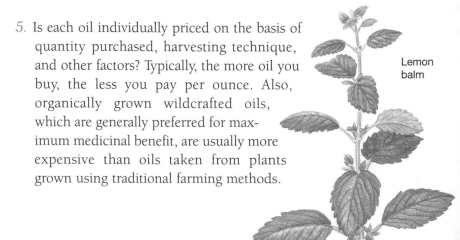

Lemon balm

6. Can you purchase a small sample of oil, or if you buy an ounce of one oil, can you receive a small sample of another? Most suppliers sell samples, and many provide free samples if there is potential for future business. A reasonable sample size is 1 ml, or about 20 drops. You may wish to ask that the sample be packaged in a clear vial so that you can readily observe its color and texture. If you love the sample, purchase the larger quantity of oil as soon as possible to maximize the chances of your purchase coming from the same batch as the sample. If the larger purchase is not of equal quality, return it for a refund.

7. What group or species of plant does the oil come from? When an oil can be obtained from more than one species, are there variations in chemical makeup that distinguish one species from another?

Proper Storage of Aromatic Oils

Aromatic oils are concentrated plant extracts and should be treated with respect in order to prevent injury, maximize shelf life, and increase usefulness. Most important, essential oils should be stored out of the reach of children and pets.

Citrus oils typically lose their effectiveness within a year of purchase. Other oils remain potent for decades, especially if stored properly. Though storage of oils in colored bottles and in a cool, dry, dark environment is helpful (I store mine in the refrigerator), the chief enemy of essential oils is oxygen, which destroys their chemical components and significantly compromises their effectiveness. Try to store oils in bottles that have as little air space as possible between the top of the oil and the lid of the bottle. As oil is used, transfer the unused portion to a smaller bottle to minimize the headspace. This retards oxidation, extending the shelf life of the oil. Plastic bottle caps are fine, but rubber stoppers can disintegrate when exposed to essential oils for long periods.

How to Handle Oils

Several years ago, while measuring rosemary essential oil for a batch of soap, I dropped the bottle on the counter and the oil splashed up into my eyes. The pain was excruciating. You must take particular care not to splash or rub the oils in the eyes. If you're using a dropper to measure small amounts of oil, you probably don't need to use protective eyewear and gloves. Nevertheless, you should follow these simple precautions to protect yourself and those around you.

Essential oils damage wood surfaces and clothing, so do not place bottles of oils on wood furniture and always protect your clothing. These oils also eat through many low-grade or thin plastics, so store them in glass jars. When you open a bottle, be careful not to let it slip though your hands and splash onto your skin or work area.

If more than a few drops of undiluted essential oil gets onto your skin or eyes, immediately douse your skin or eyes with an unscented fatty oil, such as olive or sweet almond, until the burning sensation subsides (essential oils are attracted to fats). Rest for several minutes; if the eyes or nose area is exposed to essential oils, you could develop a terrible headache. If you still feel very uncomfortable after a few minutes, don't hesitate to call your health-care practitioner or visit an emergency room.

Before handling aromatic oils, you'll want to read carefully the caution on page 25.

Aromatics for Handmade Skin-Care Products

There are dozens of oils from which to choose as you stock your Aromatic Pantry. As you learn more about the different aromatics, you can refine your collection to fit your changing skin-care needs and fragrance preferences.

The following 24 aromatic oils form the core of my Aromatic Pantry. They can be used alone or in combinations to create products to suit many different skin types and problems. This list, which names and briefly describes the oils, is followed by an outline of the exquisite aromatics I like to use to complement or enhance the aroma of these "core" aromatic oils (see page 35).

Calendula CO$_2$

Calendula (*Calendula officinalis*) has been used for centuries to treat inflammatory skin conditions, and it is said to hasten the healing of minor burns, cuts, scrapes, insect bites, and other abrasions. The deep-colored, thick calendula CO$_2$ extract is not distilled; the oil is removed from the petals by the carbon dioxide extraction method. When the extract is added to a cream or lotion in small quantities, a lovely golden color results, along with skin-soothing properties. Either the total or select extract can be used, but I prefer the select, which is easier to use.

Carrot Seed Essential Oil

Carrot seed (*Daucus carota*) essential oil is included in several recipes for products designed for mature, dry skin. Carrot seed oil's high carotol (a sesquiterpene alcohol) content gives it skin-rejuvenating properties. The oil's aroma is sweet, yet dry and earthy.

Chamomile Essential Oil

German chamomile (*Matricaria recutita*) and Roman chamomile (*Chamaemelum nobile*) essential oils are distilled from the flowers and tops of two similar yet distinct plants.

German chamomile, generally the more costly oil, is unique because its azulene, found only in the distilled plant material, lends it a blue color that fades over time. Ensure that your oil contains no synthetic azulene, which some companies use to stretch the pure oil. German chamomile oil has significant anti-inflammatory capabilities, which make it quite useful in skin care.

Roman chamomile also has anti-inflammatory capabilities and is a relaxing oil to add to diffuser blends. Although both German and

Roman chamomile essential oils are good choices for skin-care products, I prefer to use the more soothing German variety.

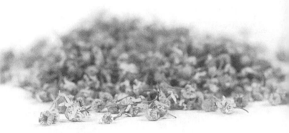

Cypress Essential Oil

Distilled from the leaves, twigs, bark, and cones of the cypress tree (*Cupressus sempervirens*), grown mainly in southern France, cypress essential oil is woodsy and refreshing. Because it is highly astringent and invigorating, I use it in toners for oily, greasy skin. Cypress oil is also said to be useful in minimizing the appearance of cellulite, though I have not found much evidence to support this claim. It is also believed to help relieve some vascular conditions, such as varicose veins.

Frankincense Essential Oil

Frankincense (*Boswellia carteri*), which typically hails from India, Eritrea, and Ethiopia, is distilled from the dried resin of the plant. This oil rejuvenates tired, mature, sallow-looking skin, while sharing its warm scent with a sweet, balsamic undertone. Frankincense is a versatile oil that creates lovely diffuser blends with citrus, wood, and spice oils.

Geranium Essential Oil

There are several types of geraniums (*Pelargonium* spp.), each producing a different essential oil. Geranium oil is distilled from the leaves of this wonderfully scented group of plants, the majority of which are native to South Africa. The premium "Bourbon" oil is produced on Réunion Island. Good for all skin types, geranium promotes stability and balance. Since it is a mild astringent, I like to use it in toners designed for oily skin. Its sweet, fruity, floral aroma, sometimes with a touch of mint, makes it a lovely addition to any skin-care product.

Helichrysum Essential Oil

Helichrysum essential oil is distilled from the flowering tops of the everlasting plant (*Helichrysum italicum*), and exploration into its usefulness to the aromatic world has only just begun. Its aroma is sweet yet pungent and somewhat spicy. Helichrysum oil reduces inflammation and itching and has demonstrated a remarkable ability to heal even decades-old scar tissue. Its skin-regenerating and anti-inflammatory properties show a great deal of promise.

Lavender Essential Oil

Lavender (*Lavandula* spp.) was used undiluted by a perfumer in the early 1900s to accelerate the healing of his skin, which had been severely burned in a laboratory explosion. Since then, it has become by far the most popular and well-known (and most frequently adulterated) essential oil, and its usefulness to any aromatic skin-care regimen cannot be overstated. Distilled from the stems and flowering tops of the herb, lavender balances and tones all skin types.

Lemon Essential Oil

Lemon (*Citrus limon*) essential oil is taken from the rind of the fruit by mechanical expression. It is useful for oily and acneic skin conditions, toning the skin and balancing sebum production. Lemon oil is a refreshing astringent, and its cheerful, lively scent is nice in facial toners and diffuser blends.

Caution: Citrus Oils and the Sun

> Like all mechanically expressed citrus oils, lemon essential oil contains coumarins, chemicals that can produce photosensitivity. Expressed citrus oils, especially lemon and bergamot, should *never* be used on the skin within several hours (recommendations range from 6 to 12 hours) of exposure to the sun; serious burns and hyperpigmentation (discolored spots) can result.

Melissa Essential Oil

Melissa (*Melissa officinalis*) essential oil is one of the most expensive essential oils, and its valuable skin-care properties make it worth every penny. Melissa need be used only in tiny proportions in any blend to soothe and tone the skin, relieve headaches, short-circuit herpes outbreaks, and relieve nervous tension. Melissa essential oil is often too expensive to use in a skin-care product. As a result, the hydrosol, which is sold at a fraction of the cost of the essential oil, can be incorporated into toners and creams to produce some of the same soothing effects.

Myrrh Essential Oil

Myrrh (*Commiphora* spp.) essential oil is taken from the coagulated gum resin of several species of shrubby plants that grow in eastern Africa and Arabia. Myrrh was used extensively by ancient Egyptians to mummify dead bodies, and it is now used to preserve youthful skin tone. It is used in the perfume and pharmaceutical industries and is said to help control athlete's foot fungus. Myrrh oil has a deep, rich aroma that is mentioned numerous times in the Bible. This essential oil may thicken markedly with age; to make it thinner and easier to work with, hold the closed bottle under hot running water (take care not to scald the skin, of course).

I arose to open for my beloved,
and my hands dripped with myrrh,
my fingers with liquid myrrh.

— Song of Solomon 5:5

Myrtle Essential Oil

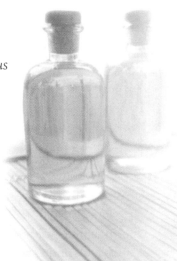

Myrtle oil is distilled from the leaves of the *Myrtus communis* plant and has a strong, clear aroma that reminds me of a mixture of flowers, citrus, and bay. Though myrtle is said to be useful to aid acne and oily skin conditions, while in South Africa in 1999, I combined it with sandalwood and rose to restore luster to my skin during the dry, arid winter. Myrtle oil has a wonderfully soothing aroma that is said to help relieve tension and insomnia.

~

Flowers do not see, hear, taste, or touch, but they react to light in a crucial manner, and they direct their lives and their environment through an orchestration of aroma.

— Tom Robbins, *Jitterbug Perfume*

Neroli Essential Oil

Also called orange blossom essential oil, neroli essential oil, distilled from flower petals, is one of the most precious jewels of the aromatic world, and massive quantities of plant material are needed to produce just a small amount of oil. Neroli flowers are harvested mainly in Tunisia and other parts of northern Africa. Harvesters spread sacks underneath bitter orange trees *(Citrus aurantium),* then vigorously shake the branches. Falling petals are collected in the sacks. Neroli essential oil has a delicate aroma that, while somewhat citruslike, is smooth, warm, and rich. This oil is suitable for any skin type — especially mature skin — and has a gentle, balancing effect.

Neroli essential oil commands a price far higher than that of most other essential oils. Thus, it is sometimes distilled with the leaves and twigs of the tree to produce neroli fleur sur petigrain essential oil. Though very different from neroli oil, neroli fleur sur petigrain is a pleasant aromatic that affords enjoyment of something like a neroli oil experience at a fraction of the price (they are not interchangeable, however).

A stress reducer, tension reliever, and anxiety alleviator, neroli tones delicate and sensitive skin. Neroli is also available as an absolute.

Patchouli Essential Oil

Patchouli essential oil is distilled from the leaves of the patchouli herb *(Pogostemon cablin, P. heyeanus* syn. *patchouli),* a favorite of many baby boomers because of its popularity during the 1960s. Patchouli is one of the best essential oils for rough, cracked skin, but most people either love or hate its aroma. For this reason, I like to blend it in small quantities with rose, lemon, and cedarwood to make wonderful diffuser blends and creams. Experiment with patchouli in combination with different oils to create blends that you like.

Rose Essential Oil

Coveted the world over for its beauty, seductive curves, fragrance, and lovely range of colors, the rose *(Rosa* x *damascena, R.* x *alba, R.* x *centifolia)* is another star of the aromatic stage and a component of some of the world's finest perfumes. Often called the Queen of Flowers, the rose is cultivated for essential oil extraction mainly in France, India, Turkey, Bulgaria, and Morocco. Its essential oil is distilled from the petals of the flowers, while rose absolute and concrete are removed from the flowers with solvents.

Aromatherapists report the use of *Rosa* x *damascena* essential oil to ease severe depression. Noted British aromatherapist Robert Tisserand suggests that this oil is also an effective treatment for aging, dry, and sensitive skin. Because it may contain residual solvent materials from the extraction process, there is some debate in the aromatherapy community about the use of rose absolute in aromatherapy treatments.

Rose blends well with several other oils, including neroli, sandalwood, frankincense, and lavender. For consistency and quality, my personal preference is the rose essential oil that is produced in the Kazanlak Valley of Bulgaria.

Rose Hips Seed CO$_2$ Extract

Rose hips are the fruits of roses, which contain seeds that are used to create this extract. *Rosa rubiginosa,* which is cultivated throughout Asia and South America, is the species used to make rose hips seed CO$_2$ extract. This oil promotes tissue regeneration and helps prevent and reduce scarring from cuts and conditions such as acne. Rose hips seed oil also reduces wrinkles and maintains the texture, freshness, and elasticity of the skin. Because of its high amounts of linolenic acid and beta-carotene, both of which are soothing and restorative, this oil is indispensable in handmade skin-care products.

Rosemary Essential Oil

Rosemary is distilled from the leaves of the popular culinary herb *Rosmarinus officinalis.* Its strong, camphoraceous aroma has a bracing, invigorating effect. For skin care, I use and recommend exclusively the verbenone type of rosemary (see page 61 for more information), which is especially helpful for a variety of skin conditions, including oily skin and scalp and dandruff.

Sandalwood Essential Oil

Sandalwood essential oil is distilled from the heartwood and roots of the environmentally threatened sandalwood tree *(Santalum album).* The most prized oil hails from Mysore, a region of India where the oil is produced under strictly controlled conditions in government distilleries. Sandalwood, which is useful for dry, chapped skin and rashes, should be treasured and used sparingly. Although the tree is cultivated in India, it may not be harvested until it is at least 30 years old, and poaching from the wild has become a serious concern. Use this oil responsibly.

The Sandalwood Body Envelope

Sandalwood is one of the most versatile essential oils and is capable of anchoring almost any aromatic blend in its pleasant, woody base. To make one of my first and still-favorite massage oils, the Sandalwood Body Envelope, add 3 drops orange, 1 drop rose, and 2 drops sandalwood oil to ½ ounce of your favorite unscented massage oil base. (See the caution on page 25 on citrus oils and sun exposure.) Envelop yourself in the Sandalwood Body Envelope or, better yet, have someone else envelop you in it!

Sea Buckthorn Berry CO_2 Extract

I first began using sea buckthorn berry CO_2 extract in 1995, when hardly anyone had heard of it. Now, it is turning up everywhere, a testament to its skin-soothing properties. Sea buckthorn berry CO_2 is taken from the berries of the *Hippophae rhamnoides* plant, which is cultivated largely in Lithuania and China. Its properties include a high amount of linoleic acids and vitamins A and E, which are restorative and soothing to the skin. Sea buckthorn berry is rich in beta-carotene, lending it a deep orange color, and is effective as an antiwrinkle and skin-softening ingredient. As such, you will find it in many of my recipes.

Spikenard Essential Oil

Spikenard or "nard" essential oil is distilled from a plant (*Nardostachys jatamansi*) that is native to the Himalayan Mountains of India, Nepal, and China. Along with frankincense and myrrh, spikenard was used by the ancients and is reported in the New Testament to have been used to anoint Jesus Christ shortly before his crucifixion. This makes sense, since the oil is said to have significant sedative and muscle-relaxing properties. Spikenard oil has an amber color and smells warm, bittersweet, spicy, and earthy. I like to add spikenard oil to products designed to restore balance and luster to dry, mature skin.

Tea Tree Essential Oil

This essential oil is distilled from the leaves and twigs of the tea tree (*Melaleuca alternifolia*) and is one of the most powerful antibiotic and antifungal essential oils. Despite its pungent aroma, it is gentle and appropriate for virtually any skin type when used in moderation. Tea tree essential oil is especially effective at regulating sebum production and has a remarkable ability to interrupt oily skin outbreaks and the flare-ups we typically call zits.

Manuka (*Leptospermum scoparium*) essential oil, a distant relative of tea tree oil produced mainly in New Zealand, can be used interchangeably with tea tree oil to alleviate greasy skin conditions and acne.

Thyme Essential Oil

Thyme essential oil is yielded by many varieties of the popular culinary herb, the most popular species being *Thymus vulgaris*. However, many types of thyme essential oil are strong skin irritants. For skin-care purposes, use only the linalol type (ask your supplier to verify the type), which has mild antiseptic qualities that are useful for oily skin types.

Yarrow Essential Oil

Like German chamomile, yarrow (*Achillea millefolium*) contains significant amounts of azulene and is useful for soothing inflamed, chapped skin. This oil is also an astringent and is indicated for treating acne, but it should not be used on sensitive skin. Yarrow essential oil can lend a blue tint to your skin-care products. I combine yarrow and chamomile to create Out of the Blue Balm Bar (page 122), a great itchy-skin reliever.

Ylang Ylang Essential Oil

Ylang ylang (pronounced ee-LUNG ee-LUNG), with its intriguing scent, is one of my favorite essential oils; I like the CO_2 extraction as well. Ylang ylang oil has a fiercely persistent, exotic aroma that some find overwhelming, and it can induce headache and nausea if used in abundance. The essential oil is distilled from the petals of the ylang ylang flower, which droop from *Cananga odorata* var. *genuina* trees cultivated mainly on Madagascar, Réunion, and the Comoro Islands off the eastern coast of southern Africa. Ylang ylang is believed to be a powerful aphrodisiac.

There are several distinct grades, or fractions, of ylang ylang oil, each named for the characteristics produced by the plant material when it is distilled for various amounts of time. The "super" or "extra superior" oil is produced by distillation of the flower petals for as little as an hour, and the "extra" fraction results from the collection of distillate for several hours after the first hour. Lower grades of the oil, which are sometimes distilled for up to an entire day, are of markedly different quality and are often used to adulterate the superior oils. Ylang ylang oil is frequently adulterated with cananga oil, distilled from the flowers of *Cananga odorata* var. *macrophylla*.

Ylang ylang essential oil balances sebum production in the skin, so it is useful for all skin types, but it should be used only in tiny quantities in any handmade product. I have successfully incorporated the oil into creams and toners for acne-scarred and oily skin.

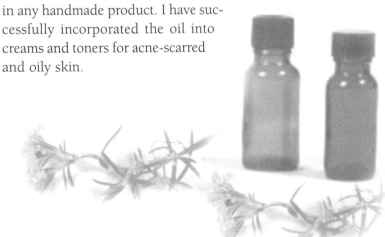

Starting Your Aromatic Skin-Care Pantry

Don't wait to collect all 24 of the oils in the Aromatic Skin-Care Pantry before you embark on the adventure of creating your own skin-care products. You can begin an effective skin-care routine by purchasing just a few oils, and you can add to your collection with the passage of time. Here are my recommendations based on skin type (all recommendations are for essential oils unless otherwise indicated).

SKIN TYPE	AROMATIC SKIN-CARE OILS	EXQUISITE AROMATIC SUGGESTION
Oily	cypress, lemon, tea tree (or manuka)	osmanthus (optional)
Dry	carrot seed, helichrysum, rose	linden blossom
Normal	geranium, lavender, myrtle	zdravetz
Sensitive	German chamomile, lavender, neroli,	none

The Exquisite Aromatics

Though all aromatic oils are wonderful in their own right, one category stands alone. These oils, which I call "exquisite aromatics," have especially distinctive characteristics. The few exquisite aromatics also known for their skin-care capabilities, such as neroli, rose, and melissa, are contained in the Aromatic Skin-Care Pantry.

What Is an Exquisite Aromatic?

Many factors make aromatics exquisite. First, they smell wonderful, which accounts for their use in the world's most famous and recognizable perfumes. Second, many plants from which these oils are extracted produce very small quantities of essential oils, or the oils are removed from the petals of flowers that are too delicate to withstand the heat of the distillation process. Because of these qualities, exquisite floral aromatics are extremely expensive and often adulterated, making the pure ones the truest treasures of the aromatic world.

Exquisite aromatics are frequently composed of substances that are said to influence human sexual desire. For example, jasmine oil contains indole, a chemical also found in human sweat and feces, which is said to draw men to women. These oils are especially suitable for use in romantic aids, such as massage oils and body lotions.

With few exceptions (see page 33), exquisite aromatics are not recognized for their skin-care benefits. Yet if a remarkable aroma is one of your goals, you would be well served to select a few of these oils and incorporate a tiny portion into some of your blends. Again, be aware that absolutes can contain a bit of residual solvent (see discussion on page 16), so be careful using them, especially if you have sensitive skin. You may wish to simply set them aside to use in perfume blends and in handmade soaps, which are washed off the body quickly.

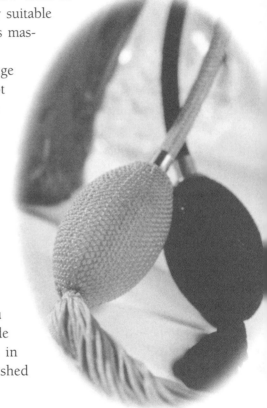

~

Like the perfumer who concocts his mixture, knowing that he must respect a balance and a certain order to obtain the perfume, we create our mixture by obeying the same rules.

— Marguerite Maury, *The Secret of Life and Youth*

Exquisite Aromatics at a Glance

You can add exquisite aromatics in small quantities to just about any handmade toiletry. Some of my favorite exquisite aromatics are listed below.

AROMATIC OIL	BOTANICAL NAME	EXTRACTION TECHNIQUE	COMPLEMENTARY OILS
Beeswax or honeycomb absolute	Apis mellifera	solvent	bergamot, orange, rose, sandalwood
Carnation	Dianthus caryophyllus	solvent	rose, sandalwood, ylang ylang
Jasmine	Jasminum officinale	solvent	geranium, grapefruit, rose, ylang ylang
Linden blossom	Tilia x vulgaris	solvent or distillation	geranium, rose, sandalwood
Mimosa	Acacia spp.	solvent	lavender, neroli, oakmoss, ylang ylang
Narcissus	Narcissus poeticus	solvent	jasmine, tuberose, ylang ylang
Oakmoss	Evernia prunastri	solvent or distillation	clary sage, neroli, rose
Osmanthus	Osmanthus fragrans	solvent	jasmine, neroli
Tobacco leaf	Nicotiana tabacum	CO_2	clary sage, orange, rose, vanilla
Tuberose	Polianthes tuberosa	solvent	bergamot, jasmine, orange, rose, sandalwood
Vanilla	Vanilla planifolia	solvent or CO_2	orange, rose, sandalwood
Vetiver	Vetiveria zizanioides	distillation	rose, sandalwood
Violet leaf	Viola odorata	solvent or CO_2	jasmine, orange, rose, sandalwood
Zdravetz	Geranium macrorrhizum	distillation	rose, ylang ylang

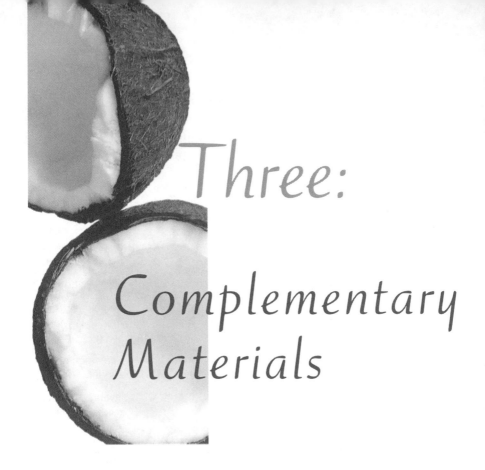

Three:

Complementary
Materials

Now that the Aromatic Pantry is stocked with your fragrant selections, let's take a look at the ways in which to use aromatic oils. Just as the stars of a play rely on supporting cast members to provide structure, harmony, and interest, aromatic oils perform best when used with complementary ingredients that highlight their distinct characteristics.

Unscented Oils

Unscented oils come from the seeds, nuts, kernels, and flesh of different plant products or from the fat of animals. These oils fortify handmade skin-care products with rich moisturizing capabilities. Unscented oils can form 100 percent of a skin-care product, as in the case of a facial massage oil, or as little as 5 percent.

Fixed plant-based oils are produced by first cleaning and cooking the seeds and nuts from which the oils are extracted. Then the seeds or nuts are processed by expeller pressing or solvent extraction.

Expeller pressing squeezes the nuts against a metal press head, creating enough pressure and heat to force the oil from the nuts. Oils produced using this method are typically called "cold pressed," though this is somewhat of a misnomer because a great deal of heat, though naturally generated, is employed.

Solvent extraction extracts oil from nuts or seeds by first combining them with solvents, then evaporating the solvents, leaving the oil. This method may leave behind traces of solvent residue. To avoid solvent residues, it is best to use cold-expeller-pressed oils when possible. Regardless of how oils are extracted, they are often further refined to remove certain solids, colors, and aromas. This process employs anything from caustic soda to diatomaceous earth and silica.

It is hard to predict the shelf life of an oil because packaging, storage, and shipping practices differ and you never know how old the oil is when it reaches your cupboard. Your nose is the best indicator of the freshness of an oil, and you should discard any rancid oil, distinguishable by a sour, foul odor. If an oil is shipped to you in this condition, return it for a refund. To retard spoilage, oils should be stored in containers that shield them as much as possible from light and air. I keep most oils that I will not use quickly in the refrigerator or freezer.

Different Suppliers Provide Different Materials

Since there are thousands of suppliers of oils and other complementary materials around the world who rely on thousands of different methods to process these materials, the chances are good that you will use ingredients processed or manufactured by companies other than the ones I use. As a result, the texture of our finished products, even when we carefully follow the same recipe, may differ. If you want the same texture every time, keep an Aromatic Journal of the suppliers that records the ingredients used. In this way, you maximize the chances of enjoying consistent results.

Apricot Kernel Oil

Apricot kernel oil, taken from the kernel of the seeds yielded by the apricot tree (*Prunus armeniaca*), is often used in hair dressings and massage oils. It is an excellent softener for the delicate skin around the eyes, mouth, and neck. Grapeseed oil is an acceptable substitute for this very soothing oil, as is sweet almond oil. Use apricot kernel oil as up to 100 percent of your base blend.

Avocado Oil

Avocado oil, taken from the flesh of the fruit of the avocado tree (*Persea americana*), is very rich and, in its unrefined state, contains nutrient-laden waxes, proteins, and minerals. It may transfer a slightly green tint to finished products. Though it also has a distinct and pungent odor, I prefer to use the unrefined oil in many of my skin-care products (especially ones for dry, stressed, and chapped skin), because it has higher levels of protein and vitamins A, D, and E than refined oil. Use up to 100 percent as your base blend, especially for extremely dry skin.

Borage Seed Oil

Borage seed oil, from the seeds of the borage plant (*Borago officinalis*), is high in gamma-linolenic acid (GLA), a fatty acid that maintains healthy skin and repairs tissue damage. Borage seed oil is most useful for dry, mature, and aging skin, and its benefits are apparent even when it is used in small quantities. Use as 5 percent to 10 percent of your base blend.

Black Currant Seed Oil

From the *Ribes nigrum* plant, black currant seed oil is loaded with fatty acids, especially GLA. Like borage seed oil, black currant seed oil supports the reconstruction of damaged skin and other cell membranes. This oil is a very valuable skin-care ingredient, and it has the price tag to prove it. Use as 5 percent to 10 percent of your base blend.

Camelina Seed Oil

Camelina seed oil is taken from the seeds of the cruciferous annual *Camelina sativa*. Also called gold of pleasure oil, camelina oil is high in nutritive fatty acids, which help improve the elasticity of the skin. Use as 5 percent to 10 percent of your base blend.

Camellia Oil

This oil is taken from the seeds of the camellia tree (*Camellia sasanqua*), which is native to parts of Asia, where it is used extensively as a beauty aid and skin-restructuring agent. Use to form up to 20 percent of your base blend.

Canola Oil

Canola oil, extracted from the seeds of the rape plant (*Brassica napus* var. *oleifera*), is extremely light in color and penetrates the skin easily, making it a nice massage-oil base when the more expensive oils are unavailable. Use to form up to 100 percent of your base blend. You may use the canola oil found in your local grocery store.

Castor Oil

Castor oil is a rich, smooth oil that I like to add to solid perfumes, lip balms, and other products designed to create a protective barrier between the skin and harsh environmental conditions. It is extracted from the seeds of the castor plant (*Ricinus communis*) and is used in vast quantities in commercial lipsticks because it's an excellent emollient. Castor oil makes hair shiny when used as a conditioner and is great for brittle nails and extremely dry skin. In addition to being very thick, this oil dries upon prolonged contact with air. Use to form up to 20 percent of your base blend, or up to 50 percent if you are making a lip balm or hair pomade.

Cocoa Butter

Cocoa butter is a well-known skin lubricant, and its natural cocoa scent is a plus for chocolate lovers. Cocoa butter is the solid fat from the roasted seed of the cacao plant *(Theobroma cacao)*, which is composed of 40 to 50 percent solid butterfat. The oil was first widely used in the United States in Hershey, Pennsylvania, when a candy maker discovered that it combined with other ingredients to make a creamy, edible substance — thus, the Hershey Bar was born. The distinct aroma of cocoa butter is difficult to overcome with essential oils, so you may wish to substitute unscented cocoa butter or a similarly textured fat.

Cocoa butter is solid at room temperature and is a wonderful additive to lotions, creams, and soaps, especially if you want to thicken the texture a bit. If added in a large enough quantity, cocoa butter may give a slightly yellow tint to many cosmetics. Use up to 50 percent of your base blend, depending on desired thickness.

Coconut Oil

Three types of oil are extracted from the kernels of the coconut *(Cocos nucifera)*. Refined coconut oil is highly processed and used frequently in handmade soap to promote rich lather. I like to use it in lotions because it adds a creamy texture and is absorbed readily by the skin. Virgin coconut oil is extracted from the coconut by use of a centrifuge that separates the fresh oil from many of the solids in the plant material. Both oils are semisolid at room temperature, but the virgin coconut oil has the benefit of smelling just like a sweet, freshly cracked coconut. A third type of oil, fractionated coconut oil, is a clear liquid that is squeezed from coconuts by use of high-pressure apparatus. It is a favorite of massage therapists since it is easily absorbed by the skin and has a remarkably long shelf life.

Note that I specify which type of coconut oil is called for in different recipes. Use refined coconut oil as up to 50 percent of your base blend, or use the virgin and fractionated versions straight as a massage oil or hair-conditioning treatment. Fractionated and virgin coconut oil can be used as up to 100 percent of a cream or lotion base blend.

Emu Oil

Emu oil is processed from the fat of emus farm-raised for their meat. It is used in cosmetics for its moisturizing effects and ability to penetrate the skin. It is anti-inflammatory and cell restorative, and it helps fade scars and ease muscle pains. Use refined emu oil as up to 100 percent of your base blend, using lower percentages for lotions and creams and higher percentages for products designed to hasten healing of burns (including sunburn), scar tissue, and sprains. This oil turns rancid quickly, so store it in the refrigerator. If you purchase emu oil that smells spoiled, return it to the supplier immediately.

Evening Primrose Oil

Evening primrose oil is derived from the seeds of the evening primrose (Oenothera biennis), whose flowers blossom during the evening and wither in the day. The oil aids in skin cell restoration and contains a high percentage of GLA. As with borage oil, superb results can be obtained even when the oil is used in tiny quantities. Use as 5 percent to 10 percent of your base blend.

Grapeseed Oil

Grapeseed oil is taken from the seeds of the fruit of the grape plant (Vitis vinifera). Though I have seen labels claiming it is cold pressed, I understand that cold-pressed grapeseed oil has a very unpleasant odor. Solvent-extracted grapeseed oil has a slightly nutty aroma and flavor, which accounts for its use in salad dressings. This oil is useful for oily skin, but you will want to avoid it if you prefer to use non-solvent-extracted ingredients in your products. Use as up to 50 percent of your base blend.

Hazelnut Oil

Hazelnut oil, used extensively in classic French cooking, is extracted from hazelnuts (*Corylus avellana*). Its skin-penetrating qualities make it especially suitable for any skin type, and it even contains a small amount of vitamin E. Use as up to 100 percent of base blends.

Heliocarrot Oil

Heliocarrot oil is taken from the roots of the *Daucus carota* plant. These roots have an extremely high concentration of water and only small quantities of the precious oil. Once removed, heliocarrot oil is typically suspended in a base oil, usually olive. Heliocarrot oil is rich in vitamin E and beta-carotene, as revealed by its bright orange color, and is packed with nutrients that help rejuvenate and fortify the skin. Nevertheless, overuse of this oil tints the skin orange. Use as up to 20 percent of your base blend.

Hemp Seed Oil

Hemp seed oil is extracted from the seeds of a very useful tall weed (*Cannabis sativa*) that grows around the world. It contains high levels of essential fatty acids, including linolenic acid, which help stimulate cell growth. It is excellent for dry skin and is absorbed quickly. Use as 10 percent to 15 percent of your base blend.

Illipe Butter

Illipe butter, also called Borneo tallow, is taken from the nuts of the illipe tree *(Shorea stenoptera),* which grows in Africa, Asia, and South America. It is similar to cocoa butter in its texture and skin-soothing properties. Use as 5 to 20 percent of base blends.

Jojoba Oil

Jojoba oil is the thick, pale yellow liquid that is extracted from the beanlike seeds of a desert shrub (*Simmondsia chinensis*). An excellent

Melody Upham, Rainbow Meadow, Inc.
Poland, Ohio

Melody Upham began crafting handmade soap in her Michigan home in 1994 after reading a Reader's Digest "Back to Basics" excerpt on the topic. Within a year, Melody started a soap-making business, and her entrepreneurial talents blossomed. Aromatherapy began to captivate Melody. She discovered that the oils did much more than just scent her soaps; they also relaxed tension, decongested nasal passages, eased headaches and muscle aches, and so much more. Melody soon found herself incorporating aromatics into lotions, muscle balms, and massage oils.

As time passed, Melody started providing a small selection of essential oils and raw materials to other manufacturers of handmade skin-care products. She also began an Internet discussion group that shared soap-making information, recipes, and materials sources. Amazingly, Melody ran the business from her dining room, no easy task with three children and a husband who insisted on being fed, despite Melody's newfound passion.

In 1997, Melody moved her company out of the dining room and into a much larger facility. What started as a hobby and soon became an obsession has blossomed into Rainbow Meadow, Inc. The staff consists of six full-time employees and the business is entirely family owned and operated.

My favorite Rainbow Meadow product is not a product at all but its unmatched, knowledgeable customer service with a smile.

lubricant and hair conditioner, jojoba closely resembles the natural moisturizing oil, sebum, that is secreted by human skin. Jojoba has an exceptionally long shelf life and is absorbed readily by all skin types. Use as up to 25 percent of your base blend.

Kokum Butter

Not to be confused with cocoa butter, kokum butter is one of the hardest vegetable fats. It is removed from the kernels of the red mango, or kokum, tree (*Garcinia indica*), which is native to India. It can replace cocoa butter, as their moisturizing properties are similar. Unlike cocoa butter, however, kokum butter is odorless. Use as 5 to 20 percent of base blends.

Kukui Nut Oil

Kukui nut oil is produced mainly in Hawaii and Tahiti and comes from the nut of the kukui tree (*Aleurites moluccana*). Kukui nut oil is high in essential fatty acids; thus, it is helpful for softening and restructuring skin. The oil is an excellent choice for sensitive skin and skin that is mature, damaged, and wrinkled. Use as 5 to 10 percent of the base blend.

Lanolin

Anhydrous (containing no water) lanolin is a fatty substance taken from the wool of sheep. Since lanolin thickens products, the use of too much in an emulsion may cause it to become sticky. Lanolin has some emulsifying properties. I typically use this oil as no more than 10 percent of the base blend for an emulsion, but I use up to 20 percent for dry-skin and diaper-rash products and pomades designed to protect and add shine to wavy, textured hair.

Lecithin

Lecithin is a thick substance taken from egg yolks and soybeans. Although not technically an oil, it can be used as one in your products.

It also acts as an emulsifier and will add a yellow tint to your products. Use as up to 10 percent of your base blend.

Macadamia Nut Oil

Produced mainly in Hawaii, macadamia nut oil, from the popular and delicious nut *Macadamia integrifolia,* is similar to the sebum produced by human skin. Macadamia nut oil is very emollient and soothing. It is one of my favorites in facial creams because its absorption rate is so high and it blends well into emulsions. Use as 10 to 20 percent of your base blend.

Mango Butter

Mango butter is taken from the seed kernels of the fruit of the mango tree *(Mangifera indica).* It is softer than cocoa butter, but still quite solid at room temperature. I frequently interchange mango and shea butter (a similar butter made from the karite tree) if I am out of one or the other. Use as up to 50 percent of your base blend.

Mineral Oil

A by-product of the petroleum industry, mineral oil is not particularly beneficial for any skin type. Mineral oil is heavy and barely penetrates the skin — a fact made obvious by the gloss left on the skin's surface long after the application of the oil. I like to use it and its cousin, petroleum jelly, in products designed for thick, wavy, coarse-textured hair (like mine) because it provides a great deal of protection against harsh winters and the pounding summer sun. I strongly recommend against substituting mineral oil for other oils in skin-care products.

Olive Oil

Olive oil is pressed from very ripe olives from *Olea europaea* trees grown around the Mediterranean Sea. Olive oil is best if extra virgin — obtained from the first pressing of the olives. If used in sufficient quantity, it may transfer a slightly green tint to products. Subsequent pressings of oil (virgin, pomace, and so on) contain far fewer nutrients than the extra-virgin variety. When combined with a lighter oil, olive oil makes a wonderful massage mixture for dry skin. Use as up to 100 percent of the base blend.

Peanut Oil

A very light oil extracted from the nut of the *Arachis hypogaea* plant, peanut oil is excellent for oily skin or for use in facials. Many people are allergic to it, however, so it is especially critical to perform a skin-patch test (see page 58 for instructions) before using this oil.

Rose Hips Seed Oil

Fabulously rich, rose hips seed oil is a staple for any good dry-skin cream, particularly one designed to heal scar tissue. The oil is extracted with solvents from the ripened fruit of a hybrid, thorny, wild rosebush (*Rosa rubiginosa, R. moschata, R. canina*), which is common in South American countries. The oil is extremely high in GLA and vitamin C and is believed to regenerate the skin and aid in counteracting the effects of aging. Use as 5 to 10 percent of your base blend.

Safflower Oil

Safflower oil, extracted from a plant called *Carthamus tinctorius,* can be used in any skin-care product, though it seems to contribute a somewhat sticky texture in some formulas. Use as 5 to 15 percent of your base blend.

Sesame Seed Oil

Aromatic, soothing, and anti-inflammatory, sesame seed oil is produced from common sesame seeds (*Sesamum indicum*). Because its nutty aroma tends to linger if used in any substantial quantity, it is at its best when used as no more than 25 percent of the blend — unless, of course, you enjoy the scent.

Shea Butter

Derived from the seeds of the karite tree (*Butyrosperum parkii*), which grows in Africa, shea butter is milder, creamier, richer in texture, less solid, and more emollient than cocoa butter. It can be used as a natural lipstick base or as a softener in skin treatments. Use as up to 50 percent of your base blend.

Squalene

Squalene, sometimes called squalane, is produced from olives, wheat germ, and even shark liver; be sure to request the plant-based squalene if this is important to you. Squalene closely resembles the sebum produced by human skin, so it is easily accepted by the skin and provides smooth, light moisture. Use as up to 20 percent of your base blend.

Sunflower Seed Oil

Sunflower oil is obtained from the milling of the seeds of the tall and radiant sunflower (*Helianthus annuus*). The oil is rich in vitamins A and E and is inexpensive enough to use in any skin preparation. This light oil will leave what has been called a "second skin" after drying. Some like this feeling; others do not. Whatever your preference, this oil is particularly useful in the winter, when extra protection is desirable. Use as up to 100 percent of your base blend.

Sweet Almond Oil

Sweet almond oil is expressed from the seeds of the almond tree (*Prunus dulcis*). It is very different from bitter almond essential oil, produced by distillation of water-soaked almond kernels to obtain an oil that smells like marzipan. Guard against confusion of these two oils; bitter almond essential oil is highly toxic and should not be used in your creams, lotions, or massage blends. Sweet almond oil is light but penetrating and is often used in massage blends, as it makes a fabulous base oil for essential oils. Use as up to 100 percent of your base blend.

Tamanu Oil

Tamanu oil is a rich, deep, thick, brown-green oil that is referred to in some catalogs simply as foraha. The oil is taken from the ripened seeds of the *Calophyllum inophyllum* tree, which is native to Tahiti and also grows in damp environments in Madagascar, other parts of Africa, and the Far East. It has a luscious smell reminiscent of butter pecan ice cream or Kahlúa (depending on whom you ask) and is one of my favorite ingredients to use in skin-care products. Use as no more than 25 percent of your base blend.

Wheat Germ Oil

Wheat germ oil (*Triticum* spp.) has a distinct wheat-nut aroma that is difficult to overcome unless used in minute quantities in any blend. It is high in protein and vitamin E, so it can extend the shelf life of other oils. Use as up to 5 percent of your blend.

Vitamin E

Vitamin E is a natural antioxidant and essential vitamin obtained by the processing of food-grade vegetable oils, such as wheat germ (it is also found in large quantities in sea buckthorn berries). Vitamin E helps eradicate free radicals from the skin, and because it retards oxidation, it helps extend the shelf life of many products. Vitamin E should be purchased only in small quantities since it quickly becomes rancid. Be sure to keep this precious ingredient refrigerated. Use as up to 5 percent of your blend.

Extending the "Shelf Life" of Your Skin

Like all living matter, our bodies are composed of a mélange of cells that age slowly (or not so slowly!) with the passage of time. Free radicals, the supreme villains of healthy skin, are molecules with unpaired electrons. Because they are unpaired, they roam freely through the body stealing paired electrons and breaking down healthy cells. Perhaps the most obvious sign of aging is sallow, wrinkled skin. You can protect the "shelf life" of your skin by making and using products enriched with vitamin E and beta-carotene, both of which help protect against free-radical damage and soothe and nourish the skin.

Additional Botanicals

In addition to base oils and aromatic oils, several other botanicals can be used to fortify handmade skin-care products. These additional ingredients fall into three basic categories: water-type botanicals and vegetable glycerin; herbs; and colorant botanicals.

Water-Type Botanicals

All creams and lotions are made with water. The variety of waterlike ingredients you have to choose from includes herbal infusions and diluted plant gels. Vary the proportions according to the desired texture of the finished product.

Distilled water. As a rule, always use distilled water to make your handmade toiletries. Tap water and springwater often contain chemicals or additives that are neither needed nor desired in skin-care products. Distilled water is available at most supermarkets, and many bottled-water companies will deliver distilled water instead of springwater for a nominal surcharge.

Of course, you can use plain distilled water as 100 percent of the water portion of your cream or lotion. However, for variety and superb skin-soothing properties, you will want to experiment with a few different plant waters, or hydrosols, as well. For more information, see page 61. Hydrosols may be used alone or in combination with plain distilled water in your products.

Fresh juices. I use a juicer to extract the juice of fruits and vegetables and incorporate it in small quantities into products — then drink the rest! Some of my favorite juices to use are lemon, grape, tangerine, strawberry, ginger, pineapple, grapefruit, carrot, cucumber, and apple. Products containing fresh additives, such as these juices, should be made in small quantities, used within a few days of manufacture, and stored in the refrigerator.

Aloe vera. Aloe vera is pressed from the thick, rubbery leaves of the aloe vera (*Aloe barbadensis*) plant. The viscous gel is a renowned skin soother that relieves sunburn and the symptoms associated with several adverse skin conditions, such as psoriasis and eczema. Aloe vera gel is different from aloe vera juice. Also, be aware that several different types of aloe products are sold on the retail market.

Read the labels carefully, and purchase the aloe vera gel that has the least amount of additives (and no alcohol) and the highest content of pure aloe. In addition, you can purchase pure aloe vera gel that is diluted with an equal part of distilled water; it is frequently called 1:1 in sales literature. Aloe vera is best when used fresh, so if you have a plant in your home, simply break off a leaf, split it open, and measure out enough gel for your formula.

Vegetable glycerin. Vegetable glycerin is a water-soluble humectant. Since it attracts moisture from the surrounding atmosphere, it's a boon in skin-care products used in damp, humid environments. If glycerin is used excessively in dry environmental conditions, it can begin to draw on the skin's own natural moisture, resulting in dryness.

Herbal infusions. You can infuse the active ingredients of herbs into water by making a tea and using the tea as all or part of the liquid portion of your formula. Choose from the herbs listed on the following pages, or select your own favorites. To make an infusion, simply allow the herbs to steep in hot water for 10 to 20 minutes. Strain, and use the herb-infused water in place of distilled water in your recipe.

Herbs

Herbs have a long history of providing multiple skin-care benefits, and there is no end to the different ways in which they can be used in handmade products. For example, chamomile tea bags applied to the eyelids will soothe and relax, while a massage oil infused with plantain, calendula, and chickweed will help heal dry skin conditions. I prefer to use fresh plant material when possible, but dried plants are often more readily available.

- Calendula (*Calendula officinalis*) — use the flowers, which are antiseptic, antifungal, anti-inflammatory, healing, and soothing for dry and stressed skin, including sore nipples.
- Chickweed (*Stellaria media*) — use the aerial parts to relieve eczema, rashes, and itchy skin conditions.
- Comfrey (*Symphytum officinale*) — good for wound healing; in folklore, it is called knitbone for its apparent ability to hasten the healing of broken bones and sprains. This oil should be handled with extra care; it can be poisonous if ingested.
- Ginseng (*Panax ginseng*) — the root is useful in combating wrinkles and the visible effects of aging skin. It is reputed to enhance cellular function and lengthen the life span of cells.
- Rooibos (*Aspalathus linearis*) — the leaves of the South African "red bush" are very soothing to the skin, especially for dryness and eczema.
- Plantain (*Plantago major*) — the leaf speeds healing of burns and wounds. It is also helpful for insect bites, blisters, and other topical irritations.
- St.-John's-wort (*Hypericum perforatum*) — the oil extracted (usually by prolonged soaking in olive oil) from the flowers and sometimes leaves of this herb is anti-inflammatory, mainly because of the presence of hypericum. It soothes many muscle and tendon ailments and makes an excellent healing agent for bruises, burns, mild wounds, and hemorrhoids. Because its flower imparts a red

color to the oil, addition of St.-John's-wort oil may lend a slightly pinkish tint to your finished product.

& Witch hazel *(Hamamelis virginiana)* — the leaves and bark of this herb are soothing, with astringent and anti-inflammatory capabilities. This is *not* the same product that is sold in drugstores.

Colorant Botanicals

Though there are a number of synthetic colorants you can add to your skin-care products, I will concentrate here on those products of nature that add gentle tints while also lending skin-soothing properties.

Chlorophyll. Chlorophyll is found in plants; it's the result of their ability to harness the sun's energy through the process of photosynthesis. It is available in powdered or liquid form and has a rich green color.

Herbs. In addition to their healing properties, many herbs can add all-natural color to your skin-care preparations. The best herbs to use are:

& Calendula — infused into a base of unscented oil, adds a golden yellow hue when added in small quantities.

& Alkanet — an infusion of this root *(Alkanna tinctoria)* imparts a range of colors from a pale pink blush to fiery magenta. Combine alkanet root with annatto (see below) to increase color ranges. (See page 93 for instructions on infusing alkanet root into fixed oil.)

& Annatto seeds — taken from the dried pulp of *Bixa orellana* fruits, give a golden orange color to fixed oils. Combine with alkanet root to increase the color ranges. (Follow instructions on page 93 for infusing alkanet root but use annatto seeds instead.)

& Fresh green plants — Plantain, comfrey, and chickweed, can be infused into unscented, fixed oils to add color. Emerald Oil, on page 64, is an excellent example of how to use greens-infused fixed oil to provide color in a formula.

& German chamomile essential oil — described more fully on page 23, this oil can add a bluish tint to some products.

& Heliocarrot oil and carrot seed essential oil — described more fully on pages 42 and 23, these oils can add a golden yellow tint.

& Yarrow essential oil — this oil (see page 31 for more information) lends a bluish tint to some products.

Leslie Plant, Leslie's Garden
Brentwood, Maryland

Leslie Plant (yes, that's her real name!) is the inspirational owner of Leslie's Garden, and just a few minutes in her presence will underscore that her love of plants is more than just "name deep."

Simply stated, Leslie was born to live the herbal life. The garden in her backyard in a suburb of Washington, D.C., is the source of her inspiration and contains a thriving cornucopia of shapes, textures, colors, and aromas. Nearly all of Leslie's toiletries are infused with herbs from her garden.

Leslie is sharply focused on activities that allow her to share her love of herbs with as many people as possible. She hosts educational herb walks through her garden, and she also teaches soap- and toiletry-making classes. Leslie offers an assortment of luscious handmade soaps, and each spring she makes soothing creams and balms for friends and family. One of her favorite springtime brews is Green Salve, a balm for skin irritations that she infuses with fresh plantain, comfrey, chickweed (from her garden, of course!), and essential oils.

Says Leslie of her craft, "I practice and share these soothing, aromatic arts in celebration of the long line of wise, plant-loving women before me. I honor these women teachers each time I handle the tools of my trade."

My favorite Leslie's Garden product is Rosita's Belize Bar, a fragrant lemongrass soap named for an herbalist who has dedicated her life to research on and the study of native plant life in Belize.

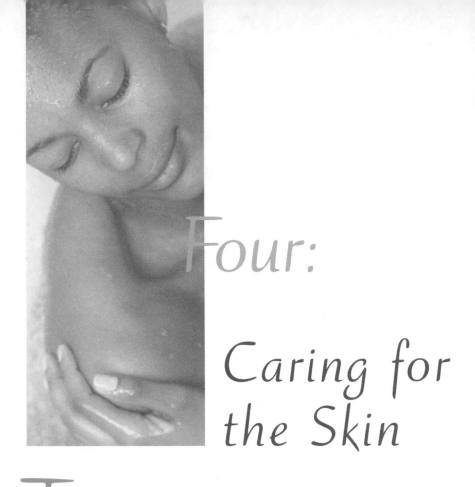

Four:

Caring for the Skin

The skin is the largest organ of the body, weighing between 7 and 9 pounds and covering an area of about 20 square feet. The skin is one of the body's most important workhorses, helping regulate body temperature, absorbing environmental elements, secreting wastes, sending tactile messages to the brain, and allowing us to enjoy the all-important sensation of being touched.

What Is Skin?

The skin is composed of two main top layers, the epidermis and the dermis. The epidermis, the outermost protective layer of skin, is made up of nerve fibers and tiny cells that are shed continuously throughout our lives. The epidermis is covered by a thin layer made up of a combination of oils and natural secretions called the acid mantle; this is the body's first defense against bacterial invasion. The acid mantle maintains a balance between acidity and alkalinity, typically described as the pH balance.

In a healthy person between the ages of 15 and 25 years, the cells of the epidermis renew themselves every 20 days. During one's 30s, the cell-renewal rate slows to about every 28 days. As the natural exfoliation process slows, the skin becomes less active, accumulating more and more dead cells on its surface. These cells are bound together by natural gluelike secretions, forming a sort of thin veil over the skin. It is this veil that causes the skin to lose luster and resilience, appearing duller and less vibrant as we age.

The dermis, located just beneath the epidermis, is sometimes called the "true skin." The dermis secretes perspiration and sebum, controls hair growth, and covers subcutaneous connective tissue. Sebum, produced by sebaceous glands that are attached to hair cuticles, lubricates the skin's surface as well as the growing hair. Thus, the sebaceous glands produce a kind of natural moisturizer that keeps skin soft and supple.

A healthy dermis is supple and flexible due to an appropriate amount of elastin and collagen, both of which ensure strength and resilience. The healthier you are, the healthier your skin will be, and it is never too late to incorporate new healthy habits into your lifestyle. Optimum health requires adequate rest; avoidance of sun exposure; regular exercise; lots of fruits, vegetables, and fresh drinking water; and a consistent skin-care regimen utilizing hydrosols, essential oils, and fixed oils chosen to correspond to your skin type.

Another Good Reason Not to Smoke

Cigarette, cigar, and pipe smoking robs the skin of life-giving oxygen and constricts blood vessels, causing broken capillaries and a host of other maladies. In fact, just 10 minutes of smoking lowers the body's oxygen supply for nearly an hour. Not even the best natural skin-care regimen can overcome the devastating effects of smoking or of secondhand smoke. If you don't smoke, don't start. If you already smoke, make an investment in yourself, and explore the options available to help you stop.

Determining Your Skin Type

Before embarking on a skin-care program, it is important to know your skin types. That is not a typo; *types* is meant to be plural, since most people have at least two distinct facial skin types. In addition, facial skin is always different from skin that covers the rest of the body and must be treated individually for maximum results. Just because you have oily skin most of the time does not mean that your skin cannot become dry, all over or in patches, by virtue of lifestyle changes, such as increased sun exposure, use of chlorinated swimming pools, and extensive airplane travel.

An important caution: As you observe your skin, pay close attention to any unusual bumps, moles, and changes in pigmentation or structure. These irregularities could indicate problems that need medical attention. If you find any unusual-looking or painful spots on your skin, do not hesitate to consult your health-care provider.

If you'd like in-depth information about the skin and how to assess skin types, I recommend *Natural Skin Care: Alternative and Traditional Techniques,* by Joni Loughran. For our purposes here, a brief description of prevalent skin types will suffice.

Dry Skin

Dry skin is caused by under- or inactive oil glands that do not produce enough sebum to keep the skin naturally lubricated. It is therefore characterized by a dull appearance and is often further sullied by flakes and scales. Dry skin feels itchy and taut and is often sensitive. It is important to hydrate dry skin regularly from the inside (with fresh water) and outside (with hydrosols), as well as to moisturize and protect the skin with rich oils that restore luster and pliability. Dry skin benefits from rich formulas containing a balanced combination of oil and water to soothe and hydrate.

Oily Skin

People with oily skin have glands that produce excess oil, resulting in a greasy, slippery texture that is frequently accompanied by large, clogged pores. Oily skin types are prone to develop acne, a condition resulting from sebum trapped inside the skin and causing the familiar pus-filled lesions known as comedones. Oily skin and acne are both quite common in teenagers, since the onset of puberty is accompanied by rising hormone levels, which increase the activity of oil glands. Despite these drawbacks, oily skin generally remains younger looking and more supple over time than other skin types. Oily skin benefits from periodic aromatic steam treatments and clay masks.

Sensitive Skin

Sensitive skin can be dry, normal, or oily and is characterized by delicacy. Because it frequently reacts adversely to environmental conditions, it often requires special treatment in order to remain in good condition. This skin type is more prone to react adversely to cosmetics containing alcohol, synthetically manufactured fixed-oil-type ingredients, fragrance oils, and artificial colors. Sensitive skin benefits greatly from natural, gentle, handmade skin-care products and treatments, including light steaming with essential oils.

Normal Skin

In normal skin, the oil glands produce sebum at a moderate rate, resulting in a balanced state — not too oily and not too dry. Normal skin looks consistently plump, moist, and vibrant. It is a wonderful blessing but requires no less attention than other skin types. It benefits from regular cleansing, toning, and moisturizing using handmade skin-care products.

Combination Skin

Most people have at least two different types of facial skin at any given time. This combination of skin is frequently characterized by an oily "T-zone" — covering the forehead, nose, and chin — while the skin around the cheeks, eyes, and mouth is normal or dry. These different types of skin call for different treatments, so people with combination skin should assess their skin regularly and use different products on different areas of the face.

Performing a Patch Test

Natural aromatic oils penetrate the skin to soothe, nourish, and protect, regardless of the skin's age or type, and contain components that stimulate, regenerate, and heal. However, the fact that an oil is natural does not mean that your skin will not react adversely to it, either because of an allergy or because the oil has not been sufficiently diluted.

To minimize the chances of an allergic reaction, conduct a patch test of any product containing ingredients that are new to your skin. Massage a little bit of the new product or ingredient (if it's an essential oil, dilute 2 drops in 1 teaspoon of base oil first) into an area of the skin where it will not be rubbed or washed off for about 24 hours. (I like to use my inner thigh or upper arm.) If any scaling, redness, inflammation, itching, or blistering occurs, you may be having an allergic reaction to the product and should reformulate it, substituting other ingredients for those you think you might be allergic to. Note that since skin changes over time, the skin may react adversely in the future to an oil that causes no problems today.

Undiluted essential oils can cause adverse skin reactions simply because of their concentrated nature. While it is generally safe to use essential oils as 2 to 3 percent (10 to 12 drops for every ounce of product; dilute further for sensitive and children's skin) of your skin-care products, you should thoroughly research an oil before using it and consult an experienced aromatherapist to learn proper application methods.

Your Individual Skin-Care Prescription

Your face is the first part of your body that is viewed by the outside world. Whether you are meeting strangers or longtime friends, your face allows people to observe your general state of health.

Most skin-care experts recommend performing three steps, once or twice daily, to maintain healthy, glowing skin. These steps may seem burdensome at first, especially if you have not previously established a skin-care routine of any kind. If you begin to follow them loosely, however, you will soon notice significant changes in your appearance that will encourage you to make them as routine as brushing your teeth. As time passes, you will establish your individual skin-care prescription, which will optimize your skin's natural strengths and minimize its weaknesses.

Step 1: Cleanse

Cleansing removes makeup, dirt, and grease from the surface of the skin and is necessary for all skin types. A cleanser can be anything from a mild soap, gentle exfoliant, or hydrosol rinse to a rich cleansing cream or foaming cleanser. Whichever type you choose, apply it to the skin with the pads of the fingers, using small circular motions; gently spread the cleanser over the surface of the skin. You can use a facial brush, cloth, or sponge to apply cleansers, but, in my experience, using the hands provides much more control over the pressure put on the skin. These items can also unnecessarily tug at the skin. When ready, rinse well with warm water, and repeat if necessary. Pat excess moisture from the face and neck.

For gentle cleansers incorporating fresh-food ingredients, try the formulas in Aromatic Beauty Food (chapter 7). Be careful not to over-cleanse your skin, and be sure to alter the number of times per day you cleanse your face depending on how your skin feels. Because my skin is especially dry in the winter, I cleanse once a day in that season, using hydrosols or a combination of fresh-food ingredients. If I wear makeup during the day, I may use a gentle handmade soap or cream cleanser at night. My routine is very different during the dog days of summer, when I usually wash my face at least twice daily.

Step 2: Tone

After cleansing the skin, apply a toner, a product designed to remove leftover makeup or oil residues and to tone and prepare the skin for a moisturizer. An effective toner will leave your clean skin feeling dewy-fresh, enabling it to better absorb the moisturizer that will follow. Select a toner that corresponds to the way your skin feels, and never use toners containing alcohol; these can cause skin to become dry and irritated. Aromatic hydrosols (see opposite for more information) make wonderful facial toners on their own.

Step 3: Moisturize

The final basic step is to moisturize the skin. Use a product containing fixed oils, hydrosols, and perhaps properly diluted essential oils to prevent moisture loss and give your skin a youthful, glowing, healthful appearance. Choose a moisturizer that suits your skin type and has as many natural ingredients — and as few synthetic ingredients — as possible.

Application of a light moisturizer in the morning, with perhaps a sun protection factor (SPF) if you will be in the sun, will provide moisture as well as protection for your skin. At night, employ a light or rich cream — whatever suits your skin type best — to give yourself a relaxing face, neck, and decolletage massage. Your nighttime moisturizer should be capable of repairing and nourishing your skin as you sleep. Be careful not to apply an excessive amount of moisturizer at night; the skin benefits from unencumbered breathing during sleep. If your skin feels very greasy when you wake up, you probably applied too much moisturizer the night before.

The Best Hydrosols for Skin Care

With rare exceptions, hydrosols have no contraindications and can be used liberally in health and beauty routines. Several of the companies listed in Resources, such as Acqua Vita, carry these items. Here are some of my favorite hydrosols and their general skin-care applications.

HYDROSOL	GENERAL APPLICATIONS
Cornflower *(Centaurea cyanus)*	Baby, delicate skin
Cypress *(Cupressus sempervirens)*	Oily skin
Helichrysum *(Helichrysum italicum)*	Anti-inflammatory uses, eczema
Melissa *(Melissa officinalis)*	Anti-inflammatory uses, all skin types
Neroli *(Citrus aurantium)*	Baby/delicate and mature skin
Roman chamomile *(Chamaemelum nobile)*	Baby/delicate skin, anti-inflammatory uses
Rose *(Rosa* spp.)	Balancing properties, dry skin
Rose geranium *(Pelargonium graveolens)*	Anti-inflammatory uses
Rosemary *(Rosmarinus officinalis),* verbenone type	Oily skin, balancing properties
Sandalwood *(Santalum album)*	Skin-cell preserver, stressed-skin soother
Witch hazel *(Hamamelis virginiana)**	Antioxidant, anti-inflammatory uses, oily skin
Yarrow *(Achillea millefolium)*	Anti-inflammatory uses, calming and balancing properties
Ylang ylang *(Cananga odorata* var. *genuina)*	Oily skin

*This is *not* the witch hazel that is available in grocery stores and pharmacies.

QUICK AND EASY NATURAL FACIAL CLEANSER

This product can be used on any skin type.

1 tablespoon cosmetic clay (I prefer kaolin)
1 tablespoon powdered oats
2 tablespoons whole milk
1 drop lavender essential oil

Combine all ingredients in a small bowl and mix well. Massage evenly and gently over face and neck, using upward, sweeping motions. Rinse well and follow with toner and moisturizer. Any leftover product can be stored in the refrigerator for a day or two, but I prefer to make this cleanser fresh each time.

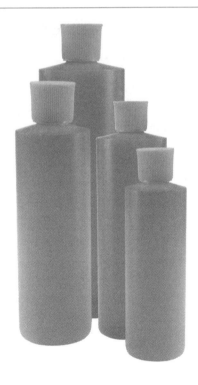

TRUTH SERUM
FACIAL-TONING FLUID

*Choose any of the seven Aromatic Alchemy blends on pages 10–13
to customize the Truth Serum Facial-Toning Fluid for your skin
type. I recommend using no more than 20 drops of an Aromatic
Alchemy blend for every 4 ounces of toner. Shake well before each
use to incorporate the aromatic oils. This recipe can also be used
as the water portion of handmade creams and lotions.*

makes approximately 8 ounces (227 g)

4 ounces distilled water
1 ounce cornflower hydrosol
1 ounce rose hydrosol
1 ounce witch hazel hydrosol
½ ounce vegetable glycerin (omit if you
  live in a very dry climate)
½ ounce aloe vera gel
½ teaspoon apple cider vinegar
40 drops Aromatic Alchemy Blend of choice
  (see pages 10 to 13)

In a clean bottle, combine all ingredients in the order shown.
Shake well to incorporate. Apply gently to clean face and neck
using a clean cotton pad; you can also rub a small amount of
toner between clean palms and then gently pat it onto the skin.
Store in the refrigerator, capped tightly, between uses.

EMERALD OIL

This simple oil can be used in any product designed to treat dry, itchy, and inflamed skin. I make about a pound of the oil in the fall and keep it in the freezer for use in handmade skin-care products throughout the winter. You can also use violet (Viola spp.) or calendula (Calendula officinalis) in this formula.

Chickweed *(Stellaria media)*
Plantain *(Plantago major)*
Comfrey *(Symphytum officinale)*
Extra-virgin olive oil

1. Collect equal parts fresh chickweed, plantain, and comfrey. Clean the plant material, removing all traces of dirt. After cleaning and rinsing well, pat dry with paper towels.
2. Shred the herbs into large pieces and allow them to wilt overnight.
3. Preheat oven to lowest temperature setting, no more than 150°F (65°C).
4. Place the herbs in a stainless steel pot and cover completely with olive oil, allowing about ⅛ inch of oil above the plant material. Place the uncovered pot in the oven, and allow the herbs and oil to heat for 2–4 hours. Leave the oven door partially open while cooking, and check occasionally to make sure the herbs are not burning.
5. Remove the pot from the oven. Strain the green oil and compost the plant material.
6. Bottle the oil and label it (include the date). Store unused portions in the refrigerator or freezer to prevent contamination from botulism, which can be transferred through the skin.

Additional Practices
to Keep Your Skin Looking Great

In addition to daily cleansing, toning, and moisturizing, four steps performed less frequently will help keep your skin looking radiant and healthy.

Exfoliate

Once a week or so, use a gentle combination of natural ingredients to exfoliate, or slough off, dead skin cells. I sometimes combine a handmade cleanser with an exfoliant to kill two birds with one stone. Avoid using harsh scrubs containing abrasive, hard materials. Instead, try No Excuses Morning Cleanser (see page 67) or some of the formulas in chapter 7 to make gentle scrubs from finely powdered oats and almonds, milk, fresh fruits, and herbal infusions.

Steam

Two or three times a month, after you cleanse and/or gently exfoliate, treat your skin to a steam bath to deep-cleanse the pores and stimulate circulation. People with oily skin can steam more regularly than people with dry skin.

To create a facial steam, add 2 drops of an Aromatic Alchemy blend (see pages 10–13) or an essential oil that suits your skin type to a quart-size bowl of steaming hot water. Seat yourself comfortably at a table with the bowl of water in front of you. Being careful not to touch the bowl, lean over it with your face about 10 inches above the water. Make a tent with a towel, allowing the steam to caress your face and neck area. Enjoy the relaxing steam treatment for about 10 minutes, and follow with a facial mask or toner and moisturizer.

Mask

A few times a month, treat yourself to a face and neck mask to balance and invigorate the skin and stimulate circulation. Chapter 7 contains recipes for several beauty masks made with clays, essential oils, fruits juices, and other "freshies" to soothe, nourish, and beautify the skin.

Before using a mask, pull back your hair from your face and cover any exposed clothing. Apply a smooth layer of the mask to freshly cleaned and damp face and neck skin, avoiding the mouth and eye areas. Rest for about 10 minutes while the mask dries; during this time, the product is absorbing excess dirt and oils. Rinse well with warm water, and pat — don't rub — skin dry. Follow this up with a good moisturizer.

Hydrate

Hydration of the skin from the inside out is paramount, so be sure to drink lots of fresh water daily. In addition, periodic misting of the skin throughout the day is helpful to replenish moisture and is particularly useful if you work in an office environment where the air is stale. I always have a mister bottle of rose hydrosol (or a combination of rose, lavender, and melissa hydrosols) with me to hydrate my face and enjoy an anytime pick-me-up, especially in the afternoon if my energy level begins to decline. To apply, hold the mister bottle about 6 inches from your face; spritz once or twice. You can even use a spray mist if you're wearing makeup — but allow your face to dry for a few seconds before you touch the skin.

NO EXCUSES
MORNING CLEANSER

*No Excuses Morning Cleanser is an exfoliator that leaves
your skin soft and clean. Grind the oats and almonds ahead of
time so you have no excuse not to enjoy this simple
pleasure at least once a week.*

makes 1 application

¼ cup fresh whole milk
2 tablespoons finely powdered oats
1 tablespoon finely powdered almonds
1 drop geranium essential oil

Combine all ingredients. Mix well and massage over face and neck, using gentle circular movements. Massage your fingers, hands, and forearms with leftover cleanser. Rinse well and follow with toner and moisturizer.

Taking Care of the Delicate Eye Area

When applying a moisturizing product to the tender area under the eye, be especially careful not to pull or drag the skin. Using the ring finger of the hand you do not write with (this will ensure that the pressure is not too heavy), apply the product under the eye from the outside corner of the eye to the bridge of the nose in a smooth stroke just above the orbital bone. Use only GLA-rich oils such as borage or evening primrose to facilitate easy application and minimize stress on the delicate skin.

RED BUSH GEL

"Red bush" is the English translation of rooibos, *the Afrikaans name for a native South African shrub whose leaves soothe dry, itchy skin. Because of this soothing quality, the smooth facial mask has become one of my wintertime favorites.*

makes 1 application

1 tea bag rooibos
6 teaspoons hot water (or herbal infusion and/or hydrosol; see page 50 for infusions and page 61 for hydrosols)
4 teaspoons vegetable glycerin
1 teaspoon pectin

1. Steep rooibos tea in hot water for about 20 minutes to make a strong infusion. Remove tea bag and discard.
2. Add the glycerin to the hot tea and stir to fully incorporate.
3. Add the pectin while the liquid is still hot, and use a hand-held electric mixer to blend. Once the pectin has dissolved, a gel will begin to form. Allow about 15 minutes for it to set.
4. To use, apply the warm gel in a layer to your clean, damp face and neck. Rest for 15 minutes. Rinse with warm water, and follow with a soothing moisturizer.

∾

There were blazing colors,
There were lovely smells.
I encountered passions my poetry can't tell.
Mere religion hadn't changed me yet;
my reverence was all real.
I remember church in the field.

— Phill McHugh, "Church in the Field"

Vicki Bedell, Essential Restoratives
Orleans, Massachusetts

I happened upon Vicki in 1995 as I drove around Cape Cod in search of a local pharmacy. My aromatic radar spotted the words essential and aromatherapy artfully inscribed on a colorful sign on the side of the road. My intention to purchase toothpaste was left by the wayside as I turned off the road in the direction of Vicki's lovely little store. Several dollars later, I left refreshed and inspired.

Vicki's love of herbs and essential oils began with a search for natural ways to counteract her own lack of health and well-being. After studying up on herbs and natural healing, Vicki quickly found herself immersed in the creative process, making everything from simple herbal salves to complex blends of essential oils and plant waters. She naturally wanted to share her passion with loved ones, so she began designing formulas for friends and family members.

After selling her preparations at craft fairs, Vicki opened Essential Restoratives, and her product line now encompasses more than 130 formulas. Says Vicki, "The love that goes into my work is as important as the ingredients. I encourage clients to listen to what the body needs and treat it with love."

My favorite Essential Restoratives product is Fine Lines Facial Cream.

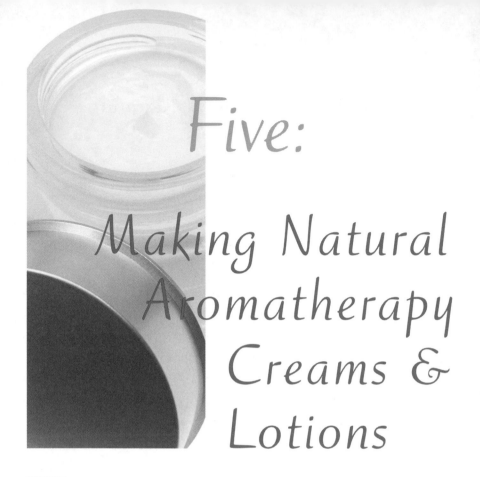

Five:
Making Natural Aromatherapy Creams & Lotions

For those of us who love making skin-care products, nothing matches the supreme delight that accompanies the successful creation of a smooth, homogeneous mixture of oil and water. We learn quickly, however, that the creation of the perfect oil and water combination — known as an emulsion — can be unpredictable and elusive. So we experiment with various combinations of ingredients in a quest to avoid the most horrific of failures: the Dreaded Separation.

Driven by the determination to avoid both the Dreaded Separation and the synthetic chemicals used by commercial manufacturers, I set out years ago to make smooth emulsions of my own, using natural ingredients. I experimented with different blends of ingredients in search of the ones that would combine to form the perfect cream. After several stops and starts, I have discovered that it is surprisingly easy to make lotions and creams that rival those sold in expensive department stores and spas.

I am pleased to share with you what I have learned thus far, and know that you will improve upon my suggestions as you make your own delicious creations.

Selecting Equipment

Take a look around your kitchen, and collect the following cosmetic-cooking utensils needed to create the perfect creams and lotions. If you don't have all of them, try local thrift stores and garage sales, which are often filled with great bargains (though you may have to clean used utensils up a bit). I have reserved a set of utensils for cream and lotion making only, and I sterilize them before each batch is prepared. (See page 90 for more information on sterilization techniques.)

Scale

A scale is perhaps the single most important investment you can make when it comes to creating toiletry items. The best scales in terms of utility and convenience allow you to measure in both ounces and grams, and are equipped with a "tare" function that allows you to reset the scale to zero after the addition of each ingredient, eliminating the need to measure ingredients into separate containers.

If you don't yet have a scale, you can use the chart on page 72 to *approximate* the weights of different ingredients.

Spatulas

Remember when your mother baked cakes from scratch and used those nifty spatulas to scrape the mixing bowl so thoroughly that there was nothing left behind for you to lick? Use those same tools to scrape every single bit of cream and lotion out of your mixing bowl. Your skin will thank you, and so will your cleanup team. I use rubber spatulas because they are flexible enough to fit around the bowl and scrape out every jot of cream.

Weighs and Means

The emulsion recipes in this book measure in grams, which are more exact and easier to work with than ounces. Grams allow you to account for the weight of lighter ingredients, so that you can make smaller quantities of product — a necessity for products that have a short shelf life.

How much something weighs in grams or ounces does not necessarily equal how much space it takes up — its volume or mass. So, for example, 2 ounces of grated beeswax by weight looks like nearly 4 ounces of grated beeswax in a measuring cup. Though it is best to invest in a gram scale in order to ensure precise results, this conversion chart will suffice for approximate conversions of grams to teaspoons and tablespoons. If you'd rather make your own conversions, remember that there are 28.35 grams in every ounce. Note: The same volume of different ingredients weighs differently. Record amounts used in your Aromatic Journal to avoid having to repeat the conversion for future recipes.

INGREDIENT	1 TEASPOON IS EQUIVALENT TO	1 TABLESPOON IS EQUIVALENT TO
Water and Hydrosols	4 grams	14 grams
Vegetable Glycerin	6 grams	16 grams
Beeswax and Other Waxes	4 grams	8 grams
Almond Oil and Other Liquid Oils	4 grams	12 grams
Shea Butter and Other Solid Butters/Oils	4 grams	12 grams
Borax	3 grams	11 grams

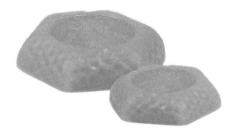

Double Boiler

This pan setup is necessary because the ingredients in your emulsion must be hot before they are mixed together in order to form a stable mixture but should not come into direct contact with heat. Although you can use a microwave, the high levels of heat often destroy many of the healing components in natural plant materials.

If you don't have a true double boiler, you can make one by placing a heatproof cup (I use Pyrex) containing your cream ingredients in a larger saucepan filled with hot water. When you place the cup in the hot water, the ingredients will heat up and any solids (such as beeswax, cocoa butter, and lanolin) will melt slowly. Once melted, they can be blended together to form the emulsion. You might need more than one double-boiler setup for a particular recipe, so be sure to have enough equipment on hand.

Small Electric Handheld Mixer

This item is useful for mixing together the oil and water. You can use a slotted spoon or fork, but the final mixture is not likely to be as smooth or creamy as when you use a mixer. For an alternative, a stick blender, blender, or food processor can be used, with the latter two being the poorest choices.

Measuring Spoons

Different-size stainless-steel measuring spoons are helpful for measuring ingredients that are used in such small quantities that they don't even register on a gram scale. Two examples are xanthan gum and borax, neither of which add any weight to speak of to a formula for 100 grams (just over 3 ounces) of product.

Measuring Cups

I do not use measuring cups to measure the volume of ingredients used in creams and lotions since I utilize gram weights. Instead, after measuring on a scale, I put the ingredients in a measuring cup, which

I then use as a mixing bowl. I prefer to use heatproof glass Pyrex measuring cups; they even hold up well to the double-boiler method.

For recipes calling for 100 grams of product, I use an 8-ounce measuring cup for mixing water-phase ingredients and another 8-ounce measuring cup for mixing the oil-phase ingredients. (Use a larger measuring cup for larger batches.) These 8-ounce containers are typically not big enough to accommodate both beaters of a handheld blender, so I use only one beater at a time to make smaller batches.

Popsicle Sticks

Clean Popsicle sticks are useful for stirring the ingredients in both the oil and the water phases before they are mixed together. The sticks can be purchased in boxes of hundreds or thousands at craft stores, and since they are disposable, using them reduces the number of utensils that must be washed and sterilized every time you make cream.

Pretty Containers

I am a firm believer that a cream works better if it has a lovely name and is put up in a colored jar or bottle with a pretty handmade label or other appropriate decoration. Even if you're not planning to get that elaborate, it is certainly more fun to use a cream

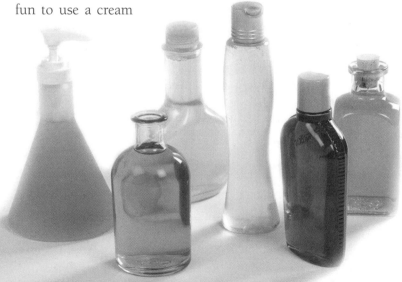

when it's dispensed from an attractive container. There are many suppliers of bottles and jars in every shape, size, and color; see Resources for suggestions. Be sure to check your local discount or value stores, too, which often sell unique containers at very low prices. I prefer to use glass containers because plastic jars and bottles are permeable and can compromise the stability and effectiveness of a product (see page 21 for more information).

Cleanup Items

Paper towels, clean cloths, dishwashing detergent, and hot water are all musts for your cosmeti-cooking kitchen. Keep lots of paper towels on hand. And since a lot of oily substances are used to make emulsions, a good grease-cutting dishwashing detergent is a necessity. When I make creams, I also keep a large pot of water simmering on the stove so I can quickly rinse off oils and waxes before washing and sterilizing them.

Emulsions: Dressing for Your Face

Emulsions are mixtures of ingredients that do not readily form an even and smooth mixture. A salad dressing, made of oil and water, is one such mixture. If a homogeneous dressing is desired, you must either shake the dressing vigorously before pouring or add one or more of a variety of substances to cause the oil and water to bind together. Natural creams and lotions composed largely of oil and water are much like dressing for your face.

A smooth emulsion, whether salad dressing or facial cream, is basically a blend of oil and water, plus emulsifiers that stabilize the ingredients and help prevent separation. Thickening agents are sometimes added as well.

There are two types of emulsions pertinent to handmade skin-care products: the oil-in-water (O/W) emulsion and the water-in-oil (W/O) emulsion. In an O/W emulsion, the oil makes up the "dispersed" phase, since it is dispersed into the water, known as the "continuous" phase. In a W/O emulsion, the water makes up the dispersed phase, since it is dispersed into the oil, or continuous phase. The more water in the continuous phase, the thinner the emulsion will be. Most lotion and cream emulsions are O/W emulsions, since the continuous phase, composing the majority of ingredients, is made up of water and/or water-type components.

The simplest and most effective way to create an emulsion is to combine the amounts of water and oil you like and emulsify them before using by shaking the mixture vigorously; this will temporarily combine the ingredients. Though this solution creates the purest and most natural emulsion, many people reject it because it is inconvenient to have to shake a product every single time it is used. Additionally, some believe that if a product is separated, it is necessarily adulterated; this is not always the case. In any event, if you'd rather not employ the "elbow grease" method to make your emulsion, an ingredient must be added to the mix to cause the oil and water to bind together and remain stable over the life of the product.

It's All about Individuality

When I opened Maria Grace Aromatherapy Shop in 1993, I knew there was a market for handmade skin-care products. My clients were pleased to purchase natural soaps, creams, and lotions designed to suit their skin types and personal preferences. Only recently have the giants of the cosmetics industry finally caught on. Based on the not-so-new principle that "every woman is unique," Reflect.com, an e-commerce company, recently launched a Web site that allows consumers to choose from 50,000 cosmetics product combinations. Welcome to the world of real people, ladies and gentlemen. What took you so long?

Creating a Stable Emulsion

To create a stable emulsion, the chosen liquids — both oil and water — must bond together as finely as possible. The emulsifiers used to achieve this bond will single-handedly define the texture of the product.

Thus, if they are not carefully selected and used in the proper proportion, the product will lack fluidity and texture.

With rare exceptions, emulsifiers are not added to cosmetics to increase their effectiveness as skin-care products. Most are a mélange of synthetic chemicals added purely for aesthetic purposes, and they do nothing to treat the skin. Commercial cosmetics companies, which produce creams and lotions in massive quantities for distribution all over the world, must add a proportionately substantial number of emulsifiers, and cheap ones at that, to their products. Mainstream cosmetics are typically manufactured to last for about two years, so emulsifying agents must be added in large quantities to ensure stability for a long period of time. Moreover, the products must be able to withstand a variety of storage conditions. All of these factors necessitate the use of unnatural substances, so that the product looks pristine and stunning from the moment you open the container until you use it up.

Choosing Waters and Oils

For your water-type ingredients, choose from plain distilled water, aloe vera gel, fragrant plant hydrosols, and herb teas. (All of these items are discussed on pages 49–50.) Because vegetable glycerin dissolves fully into water, it too should be included in the water phase of your formula.

In addition to water-type ingredients, there are certain powdered ingredients that dissolve or disperse in water but do not qualify as emulsifiers or thickeners (see discussion below). These ingredients are also part of the water phase of your formula.

Choose from the wide variety of base oils and fats listed on pages 38–48 to complete the majority of the oil phase of your product. When selecting, remember that the texture of your finished product will be influenced by the texture of these ingredients. Oils that are solid, thick, or viscous at room temperature will produce an emulsion that shares those characteristics; oils that are liquid at room temperature will produce a more liquid emulsion.

Emulsifying Agents or Thickeners

This group of ingredients facilitates the smooth combination of oil and water. Many of them, especially the gums, give a cream or lotion a sufficient "slip" so it easily glides across and into the surface of the skin as it is applied.

Acacia Gum

Acacia gum, also known as gum arabic — perhaps the oldest and best-known natural gum — is the dried exudate obtained from various species of acacia trees (*Acacia* spp.). It is used extensively to emulsify food products, most notably toffee and caramel. When mixed with water, it produces a gel-like substance that stabilizes and improves the texture of creams and lotions. Acacia gum is available in several forms. I use the powdered form and add it to the water phase of an emulsion.

A Note about Texture

The texture and color of a finished product are greatly dependent upon a variety of factors — most significantly, the textures and colors of the raw materials used to make it. Because we may use raw materials from different suppliers to make the formulas in this book, the textures and colors of our creations may differ. If you're not pleased with the texture or color of a product, try adjusting the ingredient proportions. If it's too thin for your taste, add more thickeners. If it's too pink, add less colorant next time. If it's not spreadable enough, add more gel-type ingredients.

Beeswax

Used to both thicken and emulsify products, beeswax is available in bleached and unbleached forms. Bleached beeswax is white, while unbleached beeswax retains the natural color of honey. Unbleached beeswax can transfer a pleasant honey scent to your product, and sometimes a light yellowish tint as well. On its own, beeswax is an excellent thickener, but an unpredictable, unstable emulsifier. When you want to emulsify your product (rather than simply thicken it for a balm or salve), the emulsifying power of beeswax is greatly enhanced by the addition of borax; in combination, the two ingredients form a smooth, homogeneous emulsion. You will note that in my formulas I use different ratios of beeswax to borax to obtain different textures in finished products. Beeswax is added to the oil phase of an emulsion.

Borax

Borax is the common name for a type of sodium borate, an alkaline, crystalline mineral powder mined in both North and South America. Though typically used as a water softener, borax has mild emulsifying properties that make it especially useful in handmade creams and lotions. When I use beeswax as an emulsifier, I add borax to stabilize the emulsion. Even when you use a stabler emulsifier like vegetable emulsifying wax, borax gives the finished product a more spreadable texture.

Whether or not you use borax and vegetable emulsifying wax together will be a matter of personal choice. I encourage you to try making E-Mul-Shun 101 (see page 92) once with the borax and once without it and compare the difference in texture of the finished creams. I think you will find that the cream with the borax has a lighter texture, while the one without it feels a bit tacky and more difficult to massage into the skin without rubbing. Borax is added to the water phase of an emulsion.

Candelilla Wax

Candelilla wax is taken from a shrub (*Euphorbia antisyphilitica*) that is native to the desert regions of Mexico and Texas. The wax is useful as a thickener and is preferred by those who don't want to use beeswax in their products. Substituting candelilla wax for beeswax in a 1:1 ratio produces roughly the same texture in a product. Candelilla wax is added to the oil phase of an emulsion.

Carnauba Wax

Carnauba wax is an extremely hard wax taken from the wax palm tree *(Copernicia prunifera)*. It is used mainly in candles and furniture polish and has a melting point of 181°F (83°C). It can be substituted for beeswax in the oil phase of an emulsion, but if the texture of the finished product is a bit hard, cut back on the amount of carnauba wax for the next batch until the desired texture is reached.

Carrageenan

Carrageenan is a thickening agent produced from seaweed, and it is used in salad dressings, instant breakfast mixes, and other food products. It can be used to thicken and improve the texture of creams and lotions but can leave behind a sour seaweed odor as it spoils — which it does very quickly. I prefer to use some of the other gums described here, which contribute the same thickening capabilities without the shortened shelf life. Carrageenan is added to the water phase of an emulsion.

Concretes

Concretes are extracted by solvents from plant materials. A complete discussion of concretes, including cautions on their use, appears on page 16. Add this type of ingredient to the oil phase of an emulsion to lend fragrance and a soft texture.

Floral Waxes

Floral waxes are extracted from plant materials via solvents. A complete discussion of floral waxes, including cautions on their use, appears on pages 16–17. Floral waxes are added to the oil phase of an emulsion to create a thicker texture and pleasant fragrance.

Marti Cook, Cook's Cottage Farm, Inc.
Pasadena, Maryland

In 1988, after being laid off from her job of more than 20 years at General Electric, Marti Cook decided she deserved a break, and looked forward to a life of relaxation. She was unbearably restless just one week later when, through a series of unexpected circumstances, a complete stranger entered her life and taught her to make handmade soap. Marti adapted the recipe to suit her preferences, and then began adding milk from the goats on her farm.

After selling goat's-milk soap at church festivals and small craft shows for several years, Marti inaugurated her business, Cook's Cottage Farm, in 1994. Marti now lives and works on the farm with her husband and "lifter of heavy things," Lee, as well as her bird, horse, four cats, five African guinea keats, six dogs, 30 Muscovy ducks, and 60 Saanen, Nubian, La Mancha, and Spanish Boer goats. Marti crafts a wide array of toiletry items, including soaps, lotions, bath salts, body powder, and potpourri. I was particularly impressed with Marti's goat's-milk lotion, which she says was perfected with "guidance from God."

Cook's Cottage Farm boasts a nationwide customer base. "The most challenging thing about this business," reports Marti, "is simply to keep from going crazy. I have oversight responsibility for the entire business, and I run my home as well. It's all I can do to ensure that I remain one step ahead of my competition."

My favorite Cook's Cottage Farm product is the smooth Unscented Goat's Milk Soap.

Lanolin

The properties of lanolin are more fully described on page 44. This ingredient has some emulsifying capabilities, though I would not rely upon it alone to adequately emulsify any cream or lotion product. Lanolin is added to the oil phase of an emulsion, but too much will make a product thick and sticky.

Lecithin

Lecithin is a fatty substance found in egg yolks and legumes. The liquid form is used to emulsify and stabilize foods and skin-care products. Lecithin also contributes moisturizing capabilities, but too much can cause stickiness. The deep orange color may transfer a golden hue to finished products. Lecithin is added to the oil phase of an emulsion.

Palm Stearic Acid

Palm stearic acid is the treated extraction of palm trees (*Elaeis guineensis*) and is used as a stabilizer and thickener for emulsions. In tandem with gum ingredients, it further encourages a creamy texture and pearlescent sheen. Palm stearic acid and emulsifying wax closely resemble each another, so be careful to store them in separate containers to avoid confusion. If a cream contains too much palm stearic acid, it will be somewhat stiff and chalky, not allowing for easy application to the skin. Palm stearic acid is added to the oil phase of an emulsion.

Soap

Grated handmade soap can be used to emulsify creams and lotions. To guard against adding something to your product that could dry your skin, make sure that the soap you use is not a synthetic detergent brand. Instead, use real handmade soap that you already use on your skin and without adverse reactions. Grated soap is dissolved into the water phase of an emulsion.

Tragacanth Gum

Tragacanth gum is exuded from *Astragalus* spp. (the most popular plant for this purpose is *A. gummifer*), which is part of the Leguminosae family of plants. It is typically available in very hard, dried, curved, ribbon-shaped, white-yellow translucent shavings or in powdered form. As with acacia gum, a small amount of tragacanth causes water to swell to a gel-like state, so I usually use either acacia or tragacanth (and sometimes both) in a recipe to improve the texture of creams and lotions.

Though the gel may be prepared using either the powder or the shavings, the shavings produce a much smoother gel, while the powdered preparation tends to separate. It's time-consuming to prepare the gel from shavings, but it's worth it for the texture this creates. I prepare a small amount of it ahead of time and use it from the refrigerator for a few weeks to make various products. Prepared tragacanth gum gel is added to the water phase of an emulsion. (See box below for instructions on preparing the gel.)

Preparing Tragacanth Gum Gel

In a Pyrex measuring cup of boiling water, place 2 grams of tragacanth gum flakes. Blend on high speed using a handheld mixer until flakes are fully dissolved and a gel forms. You may need to reheat the gel a few times in a microwave (on medium or high) or double boiler, since the flakes dissolve slowly and only in very hot liquid. Repeat the reheating and mixing process until a clear, stiff gel forms. Discard any flakes that refuse to dissolve completely. Place the prepared gel mixture in a tightly sealed glass jar in the refrigerator, and use as needed in formulas.

To prepare powdered tragacanth gum, use the same process as above, but use 1 teaspoon (such a small amount is too light to register on a gram scale) of the powder in the cup of boiling water.

Save Your Skin . . . and Your Money

If your desire to make your own cosmetics stems from the desire to save money, you won't be disappointed. Experts predict that by 2001, over-the-counter sales of so-called "anti-aging" cosmetic products alone will top $3.6 billion. Yet there are no mysterious ingredients in these products; it's the costly advertising campaigns, fancy packaging, and labor-intensive research-and-development programs that make them so pricey.

I have compared some of the commercial products labeled "a soothing gel with skin-repairing botanical extracts," "moisturizing honey," and "made with vegetarian food-grade ingredients" to the ones I make at home. Mine feel better on my skin, and I don't have to pay for elaborate brochures, pretty packaging, synthetic preservatives, or other chemical additives. Plus I have the pleasure of knowing I made them myself.

Vegetable Emulsifying Wax

Vegetable emulsifying wax can be either plant- or petroleum-based. In either case, the wax is treated with a detergent (such as sodium laurel sulfate, or SLS) or polysorbates (fatty acid esters), in order to cause oil and water to bind together into a smooth emulsion. As far as I know, there is no natural substitute for emulsifying wax that will provide creams with this smooth texture. If you don't want to use petroleum products, ask you supplier to find plant-based vegetable emulsifying wax. Since SLS can be drying to the skin, you may also want to ask your supplier to provide wax that is treated with polysorbates instead of detergents. Vegetable emulsifying wax is added to the oil phase of an emulsion.

Xanthan Gum

Xanthan gum is fermented corn sugar and is often used to thicken and stabilize salad dressings and soups. It lends a more fluid, spread-able texture to an emulsion, making it easier to massage into the skin.

Xanthan gum is added to the water phase of an emulsion but will not fully dissolve into the water. Instead, it should be evenly dispersed before the water phase and oil phase are mixed together. (See Step 3, page 86.)

Creating Cream or Lotion in Five Easy Steps

Before beginning, clear your work space and determine ahead of time what recipe or formula you will use. Set aside all necessary materials and utensils, and prepare your Aromatic Journal to record your activities.

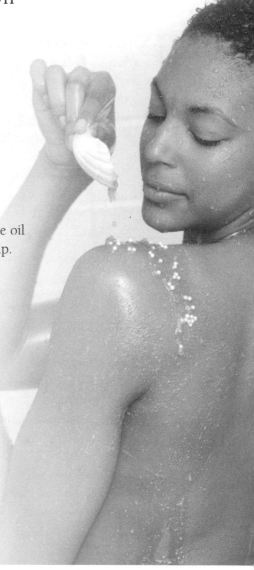

Step 1: Prepare the Oil Phase

Measure the liquid and solid fats for the oil phase into a clean, heatproof measuring cup. Measure the aromatic solids (CO_2 extracts, concretes, floral waxes) into a separate smaller container.

Gently heat the oil-phase liquid and solid fats in a double boiler over medium heat until the ingredients have liquefied. Do not add the aromatic solids, and do not heat the water to a roaring boil. Do not microwave the ingredients.

Step 2: Prepare the Water Phase

While the oil phase is melting, measure the liquid water phase ingredients (without the powders) into a Pyrex measuring cup. Heat liquids together gently using a second double boiler. When the oil-phase ingredients have completely lique-fied, remove both the oil- and water-phase pots from the heat.

Step 3: Mix Well

Add the aromatic solids to the oil-phase pot, and stir with a Popsicle stick until thoroughly mixed.

Add powdered and pre-prepared gel ingredients to the water phase. Using a handheld mixer, vigorously mix (on medium to high speed) the water-phase ingredients to ensure that the powders and gels are fully incorporated into the liquid. Most of the powders, such as xanthan gum, are not water soluble, so they will merely disperse rather than fully dissolve into the liquid. Be sure to disperse them thoroughly, leaving behind no clumps that can be transferred to your finished emulsion.

The addition of powders and prepared gels to the water phase will cause the liquid to thicken and take on a gel-like consistency. This quality gives the finished emulsion a spreadable, fluid texture.

Step 4: Combine the Oil and Water Phases

Begin mixing the oil phase on medium speed. Gradually add the water phase to the oil phase while mixing. The mixture will quickly thicken and lighten in color. Continue mixing until a smooth emulsion forms, about 30 seconds for thicker creams and up to 20 minutes for thinner lotions. After about 1 minute, intermittently stop mixing and scrape the sides of the container with a clean spatula to ensure incorporation of all ingredients.

Emulsions composed mainly of ingredients that are liquid at room temperature and that do not contain emulsifying wax generally take longer to form. Note the mixing time in your Aromatic Journal. Placing the mixing bowl in a cool (not cold) bowl of water while mixing can shorten the mixing time, but if the mixture cools too quickly, it is more likely to separate.

Step 5: Add Aromatics

Once the emulsion forms, add the liquid aromatics, such as essential oils and florasols. Mix at a low speed to fully incorporate.

Transfer your emulsion to the sterilized bottles and/or jars of your choice, tapping the bottom of the containers gently on the counter to force out any air bubbles. Use a clean toothpick to swirl and smooth the top of a cream packaged in a jar. Allow the product to cool completely, usually several minutes, before fixing the lid. Don't let creams sit for too long uncovered or a "skin" will form over the surface. Some lotions will settle considerably when left for several hours, so you can fill lotion jars fully to allow for this, minimizing the headspace between the top of the product and the opening of the bottle.

A Note about Temperatures

Unless using a wax with a very high melting point (such as carnauba wax), I generally have success when I mix the two phases together when they both reach approximately 150°F (65°C). Use a candy thermometer or other thermometer that registers at least 150°F (65°C) if you're not sure when the two phases are ready.

Although an in-depth discussion of chemical ingredients is beyond the scope of this book, some of these ingredients are not effective unless added to the recipe at a particular temperature. Check with your supplier to ensure proper use of the product.

Ginny Lee
Johannesburg, South Africa

During my stay in South Africa in 1999, one of the first things I did (after negotiating driving on the opposite side of the road) was locate the famous Michael Mount Organic Farmer's Market. Though I arrived in search of honey and fresh greens, my attention was diverted to a woman perched behind a table filled with bottles and jars. I was quickly enveloped in the scent of lavender and geranium emanating from the jars and the wooden display filled with bath bombs of every imaginable color and shape. But the creams . . . ooh, the creams. They got my undivided attention first.

In South Africa, it is difficult to obtain supplies. So Ginny Lee buys in bulk when she can, and is slowly growing her collection of combinations of rich, moisturizing oils. Ginny Lee makes her creams in small batches and stirs them by hand. She likes to use beeswax in her products, but the discovery of emulsifying wax has greatly increased the range of available textures in her line. Her favorite oils include lavender and geranium, and she makes a wonderful lemongrass lotion that glides right onto the skin.

My favorite Ginny Lee product is Macadamia Moisturizer & Skin Food.

Donna Maria's Aromatic Cream Formula

For those of you who like creating your own recipes from scratch, I offer my Aromatic Cream Formula, which allows you to plug in whatever ingredients you wish to use. It is not 100 percent foolproof, but by following it I rarely have a failed batch of cream. Since additives such as xanthan gum, borax, and acacia gum are used in tiny quantities, they are not counted in the formula, but I do count the pre-prepared tragacanth gel as part of the water phase. Although proportions can vary, my basic cream formula contains waters, fats, emulsifiers/thickeners, and aromatic oils in the following approximate proportions:

FATS	WATERS	EMULSIFIERS/ THICKENERS	AROMATIC OILS
30%*	60%*	10%	10 to 30 drops per 100 grams of formula

*To make a thinner emulsion (such as for a lotion), reduce the amount of fats to 20% and increase the amount of waters to 70%.

SAMPLE CREAM #1

*This simple recipe utilizes the formula in the chart above.
After you've tried this one, try Sample Cream #2.*

makes approximately 3.5 ounces (99 g)

30 grams sweet almond oil
8 grams vegetable emulsifying wax
2 grams palm stearic acid
60 grams distilled water
⅛ teaspoon xanthan gum

Make an emulsion following the instructions on pages 85–87.

SAMPLE CREAM #2

*This recipe has also been calculated using the formula
in the chart. After you've made both Sample Cream #1
and Sample Cream #2, compare them. Pay particular attention
to the differences in texture of the products — the result of the
different amounts of emulsifiers and thickeners.*

makes approximately 3.5 ounces (99 g)

30	grams sweet almond oil
10	grams beeswax
60	grams distilled water
¼	teaspoon borax

Make an emulsion following the directions on pages 85–87.

Maximizing the Shelf Life of Natural Skin-Care Products

To maximize the shelf life of your handmade products, make sure that the utensils and work space used to make them are clean and sterile. Use utensils that are set aside exclusively for making toiletries, and wash them by running them through the top shelf of the dishwasher two times before use, or sterilize them by placing them in a pot of boiling water for 10 minutes. I don't recommend the use of synthetic preservatives, but you can consult other books on the topic for more information about these additives.

Make your products in small batches, and pour them into clean pump dispensers and bottles with flip-top lids. Refrigerate them separately from your food in a crisper. Always refrain from dipping your fingers into your products to avoid transferring harmful bacteria into them; use a plastic cosmetic spatula or a Popsicle stick to dispense cream from non-pump jars.

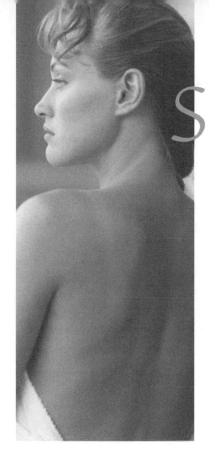

Six:

Recipes for Health and Beauty

The garden is prepared and ready to yield her secrets. Rose blossoms swirled in pink neroli cream. Olive oil kissed with golden calendula. Jasmine and ylang ylang infused into savory lotions laced with frankincense tears. Creams dripping with the fragrant aromas of aloe and myrrh. Balms to heal and protect. Sweetened with honey and flower petals. Lovingly displayed in cobalt blue, emerald green. Accept the aromatic invitation. Taste and smell the goodness of creation!

There are no rules when it comes to creating aromatic potions. For instance, you may not like the thinner texture of my Ballerina Butter. If so, add more beeswax. Is the brick-red color of African Body Tapestry unappealing to you? No problem. Make it using plain distilled water instead of rooibos tea. The only "rule" to remember is that you can always alter a recipe to create something that is uniquely yours.

E-Mul-Shun 101

*This is an excellent recipe to use for your first cream emulsion.
It is one of the simplest formulas, and has a nice texture and
richness. The alkanet oil lends a lovely pink color, but you may
replace it with any oils that are liquid at room temperature.
I guarantee you will be hooked!*

makes approximately 2.5 ounces (71 g)

OIL PHASE

> 10 grams jojoba oil
> 10 grams extra-virgin olive oil
> 10 grams natural alkanet colorant oil
> (see recipe on page 93)
> 4 grams emulsifying wax
> 2 grams palm stearic acid
> 2 grams beeswax

WATER PHASE

> 34 grams distilled water
> ¼ teaspoon borax
> ⅛ teaspoon xanthan gum

Make an emulsion, following the instructions on pages 85–87.

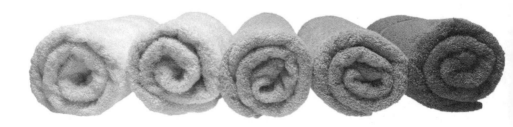

BASIC BODY LOTION

*This lotion is light and airy, while still soothing and nourishing
to the skin. The lotion tends to separate, so shake it before using.
In place of the Light Skin Serum, you may substitute
any oils that are liquid at room temperature.*

makes approximately 4 ounces (71 g)

OIL PHASE

      30 grams Light Skin Serum
           (see recipe on page 94)
       6 grams shea butter
       4 grams beeswax

WATER PHASE

      74 grams rose hydrosol
      ⅛ teaspoon borax

Make an emulsion, following the instructions on pages 85–87.

Making Natural Alkanet Colorant Oil

*This blend can be used as 100 percent of the oil phase of any recipe for
a deep, rich pink color. Use less to obtain lighter shades of pink. To make
approximately 14.5 ounces of natural alkanet colorant oil:*

  ~ *In a large glass heatproof measuring cup, cover ½ ounce of alkanet root (cut and sifted) with 16 ounces of olive oil or other liquid oil of your choice.*

  ~ *Place the measuring cup into a wide frying pan that has been half filled with water. Heat the pan over medium heat for 15 minutes.*

  ~ *Remove from heat and allow to stand for a half hour. Strain oil two times through a muslin bag or very fine sieve. Bottle, label, date, and refrigerate, or use immediately.*

LIGHT SKIN SERUM

Light Skin Serum can be used as 100 percent of the oil phase of any recipe, or use less depending on the desired texture and moisturizing properties of your finished product. As always after bottling, label and date your product.

makes approximately 7 ounces (198 g)

284 grams fractionated coconut oil
284 grams sweet almond oil
 28 grams avocado oil
 28 grams jojoba oil
  8 grams vitamin E

Combine all ingredients in a large bottle, jar, or heavy-duty plastic container. Shake gently to ensure an even mixture. Store in the refrigerator between uses.

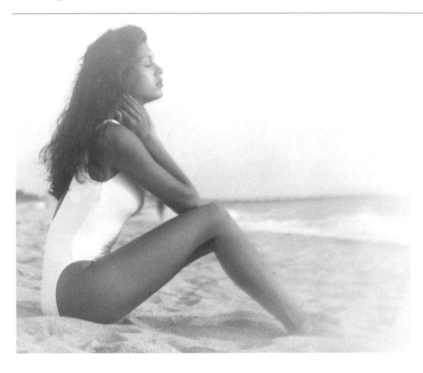

FACE GRACE

Face Grace is packed with nutrients to soothe and soften skin, and it has a lovely golden color thanks to the addition of heliocarrot oil, lecithin, and Mercy, one of my Aromatic Alchemy blends.

makes approximately 3.5 ounces (99 g)

OIL PHASE

> 12 grams macadamia nut oil
> 10 grams squalene
> 8 grams heliocarrot oil
> 4 grams vegetable emulsifying wax
> 4 grams jasmine wax
> 4 grams lecithin
> 2 grams palm stearic acid

WATER PHASE

> 60 grams cornflower hydrosol
> ⅛ teaspoon xanthan gum
> ¼ teaspoon borax
> 6 drops Aromatic Alchemy blend of choice
> (I suggest Mercy, page 11)

Make an emulsion, following the instructions on pages 85–87.

SPECIAL EDITION
SANDALWOOD CREAM

*The champaca wax, which gives the cream a slightly tan color
and lends a light aroma, may be somewhat lumpy, as it can
contain small clumps of plant material. The process below will
help strain out the undissolved plant material. You may also
omit the champaca wax from this recipe.*

*The cream is nice for dry, mature facial skin and is also good
for use on elbows, knees, ankles, and other dry areas.*

makes approximately 4 ounces (113 g)

OIL PHASE

10 grams avocado oil
10 grams extra-virgin olive oil, plus extra
    if necessary (see step 2)
 4 grams cocoa butter
 2 grams jojoba oil
 2 grams vitamin E
 2 grams evening primrose oil
 2 grams champaca wax
 2 grams palm stearic acid
 8 grams vegetable emulsifying wax

WATER PHASE

70 grams distilled water
 6 grams aloe vera gel
⅛ teaspoon xanthan gum
 1 teaspoon borax

6 drops sandalwood   OR   6 drops Aromatic Alchemy
  essential oil   blend of choice (I sug-
2 drops neroli essential oil   gest Drench, page 13)
2 drops frankincense CO_2
  extract
2 drops sea buckthorn
  berry CO_2 extract

1. Place all of the oil-phase ingredients except the palm stearic acid and emulsifying wax (32 grams total) in a double boiler and gently heat over medium heat. After the champaca wax and cocoa butter have liquefied, remove the mixture from the heat.
2. Using a tea strainer, cheesecloth, or muslin bag, strain the champaca-wax solids from the oil phase. Discard the solid material. Measure the mixture; add enough extra-virgin olive oil to bring the total back up to 32 grams.
3. Add the palm stearic acid and emulsifying wax to the mixture, and place it back in the double boiler if needed to liquefy.
4. Make an emulsion, following steps 1 through 5 on pages 85–87.

Andrea Fowler, Country Herbals by Andrea and The Soapfactory
Wyalusing, Pennsylvania

Andrea was raised in the woods, gardens, and meadows of Germany, where her herbalist grandmother taught her about plants and their uses. After earning a degree in nursing, Andrea worked for two years with a German dermatologist who specialized in herbal treatment of skin diseases. Even after Andrea emigrated to the United States in 1980, the gentle teachings of her grandmother remained with her. So when her son developed an allergic reaction to commercial soaps, Andrea formulated one especially for him.

Today, Andrea and her husband own and operate Country Herbals by Andrea, and recently opened The Soapfactory, a retail shop, on a well-traveled street in the historical district of their town. They have five full-time and three part-time employees, including an office manager and a full-time soapmaker. Women in the community earn up to $20 an hour in their homes wrapping soap, and Andrea feels good about providing a vehicle for mothers to earn a living and spend time with their kids.

Country Herbals has distributors all over the United States, Canada, and Germany. Andrea credits much of the growth of her company to the production of wholesome products and excellent customer service. Says Andrea, "A customer spending $10 is every bit as important to me as one spending $5,000."

My favorite Country Herbals product is Nature's Own Hydrating Serum.

NATURAL PERFECTIONS
NIGHT CREAM

Natural Perfections Night Cream is very rich, suitable for dry, flaky skin. The combination of rose hips, tamanu, and squalene is soothing and nourishing, and the alkanet gives the cream a lovely pink hue. For easiest application, warm a bit of the cream between your palms and pat it gently onto the surface of the skin; don't rub. Repeat the patting until the cream has been transferred from the hands to the face and neck. The rich ingredients will be absorbed into the skin on their own.

makes approximately 6 ounces (170 g)

OIL PHASE

12 grams squalene
12 grams alkanet-infused sweet almond oil
(see page 93)
10 grams rose hips seed oil
10 grams beeswax
10 grams vegetable emulsifying wax
8 grams tamanu oil

WATER PHASE

110 grams rose hydrosol
½ teaspoon borax
6 drops Aromatic Alchemy blend of choice
(I suggest Drench, page 13)

Make an emulsion, following the instructions on pages 85–87.

THE VELVETEEN HABIT

Though this smooth creation looks and smells like something that should have an umbrella, a straw, and a maraschino cherry on top, please resist the temptation to pour it into the nearest daiquiri glass and sip. In addition to smelling wonderful, this cream is a nice soother for dry skin.

makes approximately 9 ounces (255 g)

OIL PHASE

> 20 grams sweet almond oil
>
> 16 grams virgin coconut oil
>
> 10 grams mango butter
>
> 10 grams vegetable emulsifying wax
>
> 4 grams palm stearic acid

WATER PHASE

> 170 grams ylang ylang hydrosol
>
> 20 grams aloe vera gel
>
> 4 grams vegetable glycerin

SUGGESTED AROMATHERAPY BLEND

> 40 drops bergamot essential oil
>
> 20 drops sandalwood essential oil
>
> 10 drops orange essential oil
>
> 6 drops beeswax absolute
>
> 2 drops patchouli essential oil
>
> 2 drops rose absolute

Make an emulsion, following the instructions on pages 85–87.

AFRICAN HAIR TAPESTRY

If you have curly, wavy, coarse hair try this
beautifully scented, shine-enhancing pomade.

makes approximately 1.5 ounces (43 g)

OIL PHASE

14 grams shea butter

10 grams jojoba oil

2 grams lanolin

2 grams jasmine wax

2 grams beeswax

WATER PHASE

10 grams rose hydrosol

2 drops rose absolute

Make an emulsion, following the instructions on pages 85–87. To use, warm a bit of the pomade between palms or fingers, and massage into clean, dry scalp and hair, especially the ends and other dry spots. Brush and/or comb through, and style as usual.

The African Hair Tapestry Miracle

At my workshops, there is no shortage of women of African descent who want products that address the needs of their uniquely textured hair. Many over-the-counter products designed for African hair contain mineral oil, which, while a suitable hair protectant, can clog pores. African Hair Tapestry is tailored to coarse, textured hair that looks dull and lifeless (I'm looking in the mirror now!) and in need of moisturizing. These formulas are thick, and must be stored in a jar and dispensed with a clean plastic applicator or stick in order to inhibit bacterial contamination.

Ballerina Butter

To have the feet that prima ballerinas only dream of, massage this very buttery treat into the feet, heels, and ankles at night, and then cover with socks. This is especially nice after a pedicure.

makes approximately 2.5 ounces (71 g)

OIL PHASE

- 16 grams sweet almond oil
- 14 grams avocado oil
- 4 grams lecithin
- 4 grams vegetable emulsifying wax
- 4 grams beeswax
- 2 grams palm stearic acid

WATER PHASE

- 24 grams cypress hydrosol
- 2 grams chlorophyll
- ⅛ teaspoon xanthan gum
- ⅛ teaspoon acacia gum
- ¼ teaspoon borax

SUGGESTED AROMATHERAPY BLEND

- 15 drops cypress essential oil
- 10 drops lemon essential oil
- 5 drops tea tree essential oil

Make an emulsion following the instructions on pages 85–87.

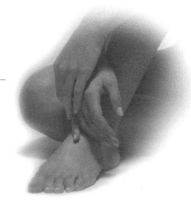

Connie Henrie
Glenwood, Alberta, Canada

A wife, mother of six children, and avid baker, Connie began her foray into the world of handmade skin care when she sought information on herbs and essential oils in an effort to treat her children's daily emergencies.

It all started when one of Connie's daughters developed a case of thrush while breastfeeding. The thrush was affecting Connie's nipples, which were already cracked and uncomfortable. When the drugstore remedies failed, Connie used balm of Gilead ointment made for her by a friend. While the ointment relieved the pain, it did nothing to alleviate the thrush. But after using a homemade preparation made with essential oil, the thrush quickly disappeared. (Connie is quick to point out, however, that she does not recommend this treatment for others.)

Connie enjoys experimenting with different herbs and essential oils to create useful remedies. Her Burn Ointment is made with honey, chickweed, comfrey, lanolin, and beeswax and has been used in several minor emergencies — including the time when Connie's daughter spilled melted wax on her arm. After cooling and removing the hardened wax, Connie applied Burn Ointment. Within 20 minutes, the pain was gone, and there was no blistering.

Above all, Connie believes in simplicity, and rarely uses more than a few aromatics at a time in any particular blend. Says Connie, "If just a few things combine together to work well, why add 10 more things just because they are good things?" Excellent advice!

NEROLI-ROSE
RESTORATION CREAM

Rose concrete and tamanu oil combine to make this cream extra
rich and special; use it for dry skin. Left unscented, it has a
slightly nutty aroma. If you share this with a friend, expect to see
her soon after, because she will likely return for more!

makes approximately 3.5 ounces (99 g)

OIL PHASE

  10 grams rose hips seed oil
  10 grams macadamia nut oil
  8 grams vegetable emulsifying wax
  6 grams tamanu oil
  4 grams extra-virgin olive oil
  2 grams palm stearic acid
  2 grams neroli wax
  1/16 teaspoon rose concrete

WATER PHASE

  60 grams rose hydrosol
  1/4 teaspoon borax
  1/8 teaspoon xanthan gum

SUGGESTED AROMATHERAPY BLEND

  10 drops Face Flowers (see page 10)

Make an emulsion following the instructions on pages 85–87.

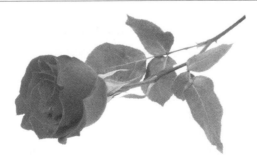

HEAVEN MUST BE LIKE THIS

Surround yourself with the heavenly softness of flowers and cream with this luscious blend of nutrients designed to treat dry skin. This lotion is very smooth and spreads easily onto your clean, damp face, neck, and body after a warm bath.

makes approximately 4 ounces (113 g)

OIL PHASE

12 grams avocado oil
10 grams extra-virgin olive oil
8 grams vegetable emulsifying wax
6 grams cocoa butter
2 grams vitamin E
2 grams jojoba oil
6 grams stearic acid

WATER PHASE

40 grams rose hydrosol
36 grams neroli hydrosol

SUGGESTED AROMATHERAPY BLEND

10 drops Face Flowers (see page 10)

Make an emulsion following the instructions on pages 85–87.

Baldini emerged from his laboratory almost daily with some new scent. And what scents they were! Not just perfumes of high, indeed highest quality, but also cremes, powders, soaps, hair tonics, toilet waters, oils . . . Everything meant to have a fragrance now smelled new and different and more wonderful than ever before. As if bewitched, the public pounced upon everything, absolutely everything — even the newfangled scented chair ribbons that Baldini crafted one day on a curious whim.

— Patrick Süskind, *Perfume*

HELPING HAND CREAM

A lovely cream to soothe dryness, Helping Hand Cream is loaded with richness to help heal even the most mistreated skin. Use nightly for best results.

makes approximately 2 ounces (57 g)

OIL PHASE

    10 grams avocado oil
    10 grams shea butter
     4 grams beeswax
     6 grams lanolin

WATER PHASE

    24 grams melissa hydrosol
     2 grams grated handmade soap (if you don't want to make your own, try Leslie's Garden's Easy Soap)

SUGGESTED AROMATHERAPY BLEND

     8 drops Mercy (see page 11)

Make an emulsion, following the instructions on pages 85–87.

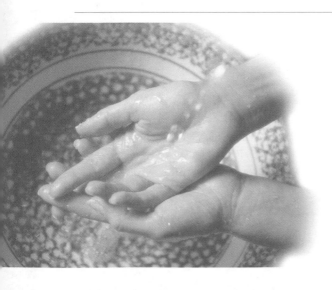

SHEA BUTTER CREAM

At the 1998 Aromatic Girlfriend Party, what a time we had shar-
ing handmade treats and sampling the exquisite aromatics pro-
vided by Rachael Shapiro, from A Woman of Uncommon Scents.
I made everyone a jar of Shea Butter Cream, each scented with
a few drops of the world's best aromatics. I just love being a girl!

makes approximately 4 ounces (113 g)

OIL PHASE

18 grams extra-virgin olive oil
16 grams shea butter
10 grams vegetable emulsifying wax
2 grams orange wax
2 grams palm stearic acid

WATER PHASE

40 grams rose hydrosol
20 grams rose geranium hydrosol
1 teaspoon borax
⅛ teaspoon xanthan gum

SUGGESTED AROMATHERAPY BLEND

15 drops Face Flowers (see page 10)

Make an emulsion, following the instructions on pages 85–87.

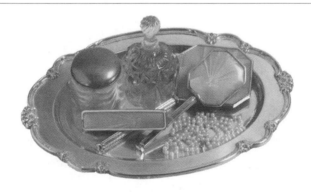

Golden Flowers

With a golden color and fragrance from the rarest petals, Golden Flowers is a wonderful cream for nourishing and soothing dry skin.

makes approximately 4 ounces (113 g)

Oil Phase

10 grams emulsifying wax

8 grams rose hips seed oil

6 grams heliocarrot oil

6 grams avocado oil

6 grams tamanu oil

4 grams St.-John's-wort oil

4 grams neroli wax

4 grams camellia oil

Water Phase

20 grams neroli hydrosol

20 grams rose hydrosol

10 grams rose geranium hydrosol

8 grams prepared tragacanth gel (see page 83)

Suggested Aromatherapy Blend

15 drops Face Flowers (see page 10)

Make an emulsion, following the instructions on pages 85–87.

Caring for Your Hands

For a lifetime of beautiful hands and nails, do not expose them to sunlight, especially during the hottest times of the day. Wear gloves to perform daily housecleaning rituals. Use Many Splendid Things cuticle balm (see page 120) and Helping Hand Cream (see page 106) regularly.

DESSERT FOR YOUR SKIN

Dessert for Your Skin body lotion feels like soft mousse.
Made with soothing rooibos tea, this lotion is suitable
for normal and dry skin alike.

makes approximately 9 ounces (255 g)

OIL PHASE

    62 grams refined coconut oil
    30 grams Dry Skin Blend
      (see formula on page 112)
    20 grams shea butter
    10 grams beeswax
    14 grams palm stearic acid

WATER PHASE

    110 grams rooibos tea
    16 grams vegetable glycerin
    4 grams borax

SUGGESTED AROMATHERAPY BLEND

    4 grams Drench (see page 13)

Make an emulsion, following the instructions on pages 85–87.

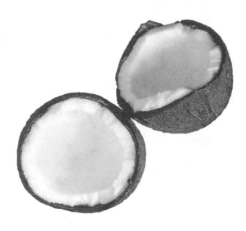

African Body Tapestry

This brick-red lotion is a favorite to soothe any wintertime skin, but I like to make it for my African "sisters," who love the rich texture and emollient character. (My friend Jennifer calls this her "wonderful black girl's lotion.") How fitting that it should include a healthy dose of a native South African herb, rooibos, said to ease symptoms of eczema. Although I suggest an aromatic blend, you can also leave the lotion unscented and enjoy the light natural scent of rooibos and virgin coconut oil.

makes approximately 10 ounces (284 g)

Oil Phase

- 62 grams refined coconut oil
- 56 grams extra-virgin olive oil
- 20 grams virgin coconut oil
- 12 grams beeswax
- 4 grams cocoa butter
- 4 grams shea butter
- 4 grams palm stearic acid

Water Phase

- 100 grams rooibos tea (see step 1)
- 20 grams vegetable glycerin
- 4 grams borax
- 4 grams prepared tragacanth gel (see page 83)

Suggested Aromatherapy Blend

- 10 grams Drench (see page 13)

1. Make a rooibos infusion by steeping two tea bags in 100 grams of hot distilled water.
2. Make an emulsion, following the instructions on pages 85–87.

PUNCH LINES FACIAL CREAM

Give those lines a TKO with this lovely peach-colored cream, inspired by a recipe developed at an Aromatic Beauty Workshop. It glides smoothly onto the skin and is absorbed quickly and completely, making it appropriate for dry skin, too. Pretty in peach!

makes approximately 7 ounces (198 g)

OIL PHASE

> 22 grams sweet almond oil
>
> 16 grams avocado oil
>
> 16 grams vegetable emulsifying wax
>
> 10 grams jojoba oil
>
> 4 grams macadamia nut oil
>
> 4 grams heliocarrot oil
>
> 4 grams natural alkanet colorant oil (see page 93)
>
> 4 grams palm stearic acid

WATER PHASE

> 116 grams melissa hydrsol
>
> 6 grams prepared tragacanth gel (see page 83)
>
> ¼ teaspoon acacia gum

SUGGESTED AROMATHERAPY BLEND

> 3 grams Drench (see page 13)

Make an emulsion, following the instructions on pages 85–87.

Dry Skin Blend

*Use this blend as 100 percent of the oil phase of any recipe,
or use less depending on the desired texture and moisturizing
properties of your finished product. Because of the calendula
and carrot oils, Dry Skin Blend can add a slightly orange
or golden color to your finished product.*

makes approximately 7 ounces (198 g)

85 grams sweet almond oil
42 grams jojoba oil
42 grams avocado oil
4 grams wheat germ oil
6 grams rose hips seed oil
4 grams borage seed oil
4 grams evening primrose oil
4 grams foraha oil
4 grams heliocarrot oil
4 grams calendula-infused oil (available through
   some of the suppliers listed in Resources)

Combine all ingredients in a large, clean bottle, jar, or heavy-duty
plastic container. Shake gently to ensure an even mixture. Store in
the refrigerator between uses.

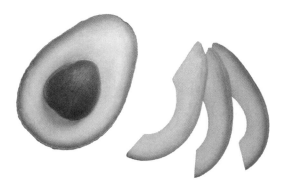

BLESSINGWAY CREAM

*Some Native American cultures call for a blessingway ceremony
in which the entire community celebrates the upcoming birth
of a baby. Gently smoothing Blessingway Cream over
the stretching belly skin of a mother-to-be is soothing
and nurturing for her and the baby.*

makes approximately 5 ounces (142 g)

OIL PHASE

    28 grams cocoa butter
    16 grams extra-virgin olive oil
    8 grams vegetable emulsifying wax
    4 grams mango butter
    2 grams shea butter
    2 grams sweet almond oil
    2 grams wheat germ oil
    2 grams palm stearic acid

WATER PHASE

    84 grams neroli hydrosol
    ½ teaspoon xanthan gum
    ½ teaspoon borax

Make an emulsion, following the instructions on pages 85–87.

*When the soul approaches the mysteries; when it tries to rally to the great spiritual
principles, the perfumes are there. The odor of incense and roses fills the temples
and churches of every religion in the world.*

— Marguerite Maury, *The Secret of Life and Youth*

Second Skin Elixirs

There is, of course, great value in a product containing moisture-rich oils, skin-loving plant waters, and pure essential oils. But what about the value of emulsifiers or thickeners? Let's face it, as much as the addition of these ingredients increases the aesthetic appeal of a product, it does nothing to treat the skin. I now share with you my recipes for Second Skin Elixirs, silky-smooth formulas that contain no emulsifiers, no gums, and no thickeners, and are easily absorbable and 100 percent nourishing. If care is taken to choose ingredients suited for your skin type, they are indeed the purest form of skin-soothing emulsion. (You can also try making your favorite emulsion formula without the thickeners and waxes, and adjust the proportion of oil and water to account for your personal preferences — I recommend a blend of 50 percent oil to 50 percent water.)

Store Second Skin Elixir in the refrigerator. I store mine in an amber bottle with a screw top, and since rubber can degrade aromatic oils, I keep a dropper nearby to dispense about 1 dropperful for a face and neck application. I can easily use a half ounce if I am treating my whole body. Remember to shake well before using.

MELISSA–ROSE

This special elixir is for normal to dry skin.

makes approximately 1 ounce (28 g)

14 grams rose hydrosol
10 grams rose hips seed oil
4 grams camellia oil
2 drops rose essential oil
1 drop melissa essential oil

Put all ingredients in a clean 1-ounce bottle. Cap and shake gently to ensure an even mixture. Dispense with a pipette or glass dropper.

DRY SKIN SUNDAE

Dry Skin Sundae is truly a treat for dry skin.

makes approximately 1 ounce (28 g)

16 grams rose geranium hydrosol
4 grams avocado oil
4 grams rose hips seed oil
4 grams camelina seed oil
2 drops rose essential oil
1 drop patchouli essential oil

Put all ingredients in a clean 1-ounce bottle. Cap and shake gently to ensure an even mixture. Dispense with a pipette or glass dropper.

DEW DROP

If you have normal skin, you'll love this recipe.

makes approximately 1 ounce (28 g)

14 grams rose hydrosol
8 grams sweet almond oil
6 grams jojoba oil
4 drops geranium essential oil
2 drops lavender essential oil
1 drop ylang ylang essential oil

Put all ingredients in a clean 1-ounce bottle. Cap and shake gently to ensure an even mixture. Dispense with a pipette or glass dropper.

AbraCaDaBra

A fantastically rich lotion, this skin elixir may help fade scar tissue.

makes approximately 1 ounce (28 g)

12 grams emu oil

10 grams helichrysum hydrosol

2 grams tamanu oil

6 drops CO_2 Crew (see page 10)

6 drops Face Flowers or Mercy Aromatic Alchemy blend (see pages 10, 11)

Put all ingredients in a clean 1-ounce bottle. Cap and shake gently to ensure an even mixture. Dispense with a pipette or glass dropper.

Soothe

Don't suffer from itchy, inflamed skin; try this remedy instead.

makes approximately 1 ounce (28 g)

12 grams yarrow hydrosol

12 grams Emerald Oil (see page 64)

2 grams emu oil

6 drops Mercy Aromatic Alchemy blend (see page 11)

Put all ingredients in a clean 1-ounce bottle. Cap and shake gently to ensure an even mixture. Dispense with a pipette or glass dropper.

GRACEFUL

Give maturing skin a boost with this lavishly scented lotion.

makes approximately 1 ounce (28 g)

18 grams sandalwood hydrosol or neroli hydrosol
8 grams rose hips seed oil
2 grams evening primrose oil (or black currant
seed oil or borage seed oil)
2 drops carrot seed essential oil
2 drops myrrh essential oil
1 drop frankincense essential oil

Put all ingredients in a clean 1-ounce bottle. Cap and shake gently to mix. Dispense with a pipette or glass dropper.

YOU BLOOM GIRL!

This recipe is for normal to oily skin.

makes approximately 1 ounce (28 g)

14 grams cypress hydrosol
4 grams hazelnut oil
4 grams jojoba oil
4 grams grapeseed oil
1 drop sandalwood essential oil
1 drop geranium essential oil
1 drop rose essential oil
1 drop lavender essential oil

Put all ingredients in a clean 1-ounce bottle. Cap and shake gently to ensure an even mixture. Dispense with a pipette or glass dropper.

Lip and Nail Balms

These buttery beauty items are mixtures of oils and waxes, which thicken together to form healthy "food" for nails and lips. When making these balms, be sure to use a mixing cup with a pour spout so that you can easily pour the product into small tubes or jars.

ALL THAT JAZZMIN

This is an especially fragrant balm with a transparent pink-brown color infused with ingredients that fortify and soothe.

makes approximately 1 ounce (28 g), or four .25-ounce lip balm tubes or two ½-ounce jars

6 grams jojoba oil
6 grams natural alkanet colorant oil (see page 93)
4 grams tamanu oil
4 grams rose hips seed oil
4 grams beeswax
3 grams jasmine wax (or 3 more grams of beeswax)
4 drops sea buckthorn berry CO_2
2 drops jasmine absolute

1. Put all ingredients except the jasmine absolute and sea buckthorn berry in a mixing cup. Using the double-boiler method (page 73), heat until almost all wax is melted.
2. Remove from heat and stir with a Popsicle stick to melt and incorporate the remainder of the wax. When the wax has completely melted, add jasmine absolute and sea buckthorn berry CO_2. Stir to mix.
3. Carefully transfer into lip balm tubes or jars.

LIP TANGO IN PARADISE

Smooth and sultry. Soft and supple. Your lips can be all of these things and more if you use Lip Tango in Paradise. You'll want to take this soothing mixture of oils bathed in the scent of honey and jasmine with you everywhere. Note: *You may substitute beeswax for the jasmine wax. You may also substitute 1 teaspoon of honey-scented fragrance oil for the beeswax absolute.*

makes approximately 2.5 ounces (71 g), or ten .25-ounce lip balm tubes

1 ounce olive oil
.3 ounce lanolin
.4 ounce almond oil
.3 ounce natural alkanet colorant oil (see page 93)
.3 ounce beeswax
.1 ounce jasmine wax
5 drops beeswax absolute

1. Carefully measure all ingredients except the beeswax absolute into your mixing cup. Using the double-boiler method (see page 73), heat the ingredients until almost all wax is melted.
2. Remove from heat and stir with a Popsicle stick to melt the remainder of the wax and incorporate. When the wax has completely melted, add beeswax absolute and stir to mix.
3. Carefully transfer into lip balm tubes or jars.

MANY SPLENDID THINGS

*During the wintertime, the skin around my fingernails
used to become dry, cracked, and very ugly. So I decided to put
many splendid things in a pot and stir them up together. This
product is the wonderful result, with some of the best skin-care
oils to soothe and nourish the cuticles and skin around the nail
bed, and essential oils to protect against nail fungus. A friend
of mine swears her nails grow faster when she uses this!
You may substitute beeswax for the carnauba wax.
You may also substitute any rich oil for the Dry Skin Blend
(see pages 114–116 for selections).*

makes approximately 2.5 ounces (71 g)

1 ounce Dry Skin Blend (see page 112)
.7 ounce jojoba oil
.3 ounce lanolin
.5 ounce carnauba wax
10 drops each lemon and frankincense
   essential oils
5 drops tea tree essential oil

1. Carefully measure all ingredients except the essential oils into your mixing cup. Using the double-boiler method (see page 73), heat the ingredients until almost all the wax is melted.
2. Remove from heat and stir with a Popsicle stick to melt and incorporate the remainder of the wax. When the wax has completely melted, add essential oils and stir to mix.
3. Carefully transfer into clean jars.

Donna Maria's Balm Bars

Lately, moisturizing combinations of oils and waxes called lotion bars have become quite popular. These products are very similar to lip balms, only they are molded into easy-to-use shapes so they can be held and massaged over the surface of the skin. "Lotion bar" is a misnomer, since lotions are really emulsions of oil and water, and lotion bars contain no water. To avoid confusion, I call these wonderful skin-soothing treats Balm Bars, and here are some of my favorites.

To make Balm Bars:

1. Melt the ingredients together in a double boiler, adding the aromatics last. (You can substitute scented or unscented cocoa butter for any of the butters, but scented cocoa butter will substantially change the aroma.)

2. Stir well to incorporate, and pour into molds sized to fit comfortably into your palm. Try using clean candy molds, ice-cube trays, toiletries molds, or other small plastic containers. You can also pour the mixture into push-up containers, like those used for deodorants. These containers are more convenient, since you can apply the balm directly from its holder.

3. Place Balm Bars in the freezer for about 20 minutes. Balm Bars should be refrigerated between uses to help maintain their shape and texture. I store my Balm Bars in clean yogurt containers. Wrap them in pretty paper or cloth if they are gifts.

OUT OF THE BLUE BALM BAR

Made green by Emerald Oil, German chamomile, and yarrow, this balm bar will soothe and nourish itchy, chapped skin.

30 grams kokum butter
30 grams Emerald Oil (see page 64)
24 grams beeswax
8 grams mango butter
2 grams yarrow essential oil
2 grams German chamomile essential oil

Follow directions for making Balm Bars on page 121. To use, first warm the bar gently between your palms so that the balm transfers to your hands. Apply the balm to your skin with your palms. You can also massage the bar directly onto the skin. If you're using a push-up container, simply apply the balm directly from the container to your skin.

VANILLA NECTAR BALM BAR

This Balm Bar is made golden by the addition of heliocarrot, annatto, and the CO_2 Crew. Use it to moisturize dry, flaky skin.

30 grams illipe butter
30 grams beeswax
26 grams natural annatto colorant oil (make like the alkanet oil, page 93, but with annatto)
4 grams heliocarrot oil
4 grams vanilla absolute
2 grams CO_2 Crew (see page 10)

Follow directions for making Balm Bars on page 121. See the directions for use in the recipe above.

GIRL CURVES BALM BAR

Tend to your beautiful curves with this fuchsia-colored treat that incorporates alkanet, annatto, and rose concrete.

30 grams shea butter
30 grams beeswax
16 grams natural alkanet colorant oil (page 93)
14 grams natural annatto colorant oil (make like the alkanet oil, page 93, but with annatto)
6 grams orange wax
1/16 teaspoon rose concrete

Follow directions for making Balm Bars on page 121. See the directions for use in the recipe on the previous page.

ABRACADABRA BALM BAR

Scars are created when, following surgery, a wound, or other invasive activity, connective tissue accumulates on the skin's surface. Regular use of this formula can help fade even old scars.

40 grams beeswax
30 grams shea butter
20 grams emu oil
10 grams tamanu oil
6 grams lanolin
4 grams walnut oil
10 drops helichrysum essential oil
10 drops lavender essential oil
6 drops German chamomile essential oil

Follow directions for making Balm Bars on page 121. See the directions for use in the recipe on the previous page.

Pat Silver
Bristol, England

Pat Silver lives in a village in southwestern England with her partner, Dave, two Bengal cats, and a garden filled with herbs and "a whole host of weeds."

Pat is a jill-of-all-trades, if ever there was one. She is a classical guitarist, singer, herb grower, backpacker, needleworker, radio technician, National Herb Society member, and student at the National Institute of Medicinal Herbalists. Pat also finds time to combine her chemistry and botany training with her love for plants to create skincare products for loved ones. If all that wasn't enough to distinguish Pat, in 1998 the traditional Japanese Christmas tree ornament she embroidered was selected by members of the British Royal School of Needlework and displayed on the Queen's Christmas tree!

Pat's toiletries adventures began when she ran out of her commercial gardener's cream. Rather than purchase another jar, she decided to try making her own. The simple combination of olive oil, water, and beeswax worked wonders for her skin, and the success prompted her to try making lotions, bath salts, and lip balms.

According to Pat, "Knowledge is of no practical use unless it is shared. In our technological world, I think it is empowering to learn how to be self-sufficient even if only in a small way." In that spririt of sharing, Pat graciously allowed me to pass along one of her favorite recipes, Chickweed Cream for Minor Skin Irritations (next page). Naturally, it's a favorite!

PAT SILVER'S CHICKWEED CREAM FOR MINOR SKIN IRRITATIONS

This simple recipe soothes skin problems, including eczema, dry rashes, and itching. In the past, an herbalist would have simply added chopped chickweed to a solid fat, such as lard, warmed the lard until it turned green, strained the herb-infused liquid, and used it as an ointment. That would still be effective, but it's much nicer to use a basic cream recipe, adding lavender essential oil.

makes 3 ounces (85 g)

2 tablespoons chickweed infusion
¼ teaspoon borax (or pure handmade soap; if you don't want to make your own, try Woodspirits' Lamb Cakes)
2 tablespoons almond oil (or other light oil)
1 teaspoon lanolin (for very dry skin only)
2 teaspoons grated beeswax
2 drops lavender essential oil (optional)

1. To prepare chickweed infusion, thoroughly wash a handful of fresh chickweed, trimming off roots and yellow leaves. Finely chop and just cover with boiling water. Set aside to cool. When cool, mash the chickweed. Strain.
2. Dissolve the borax or soap in the chickweed infusion, warming it if necessary over low heat.
3. Warm the oil, lanolin (if used), and wax over low heat until the wax has melted. Making sure that both the oils and infusion are at about the same temperature, pour the infusion slowly into the oils, beating all the time until it starts to thicken.
4. Stir in the lavender essential oil. Pour the mixture into small pots. Store in the refrigerator.

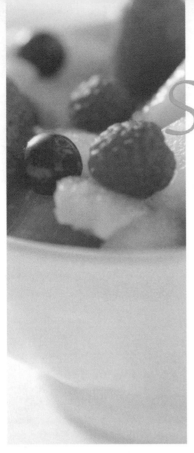

Seven:

Aromatic Beauty Food

*U*sing fresh, natural products from the earth to honor our bodies is one of the highest forms of praise we can express, and one of the most beautiful. The earth's bountiful yield of succulent fruits and vegetables provides us with the means to pamper ourselves with the pure and natural every day. How blessed we are to have access to these fresh gifts from the ground! There's almost no excuse for not enjoying them as frequently as possible.

When I feel stressed out and overwhelmed, by either work or some self-imposed pressure, taking just 5 or 10 minutes to enjoy a luscious pear or a juicy slice of cantaloupe is all I need to calm and soothe me. My senses of sight, smell, and taste interact with the texture of the food in my mouth to create a sensual and pleasurable feast. Several deep breaths between each bite help me to slow down and really enjoy the food and be thankful for its provision.

Fruit on Your Face?

Though the sweet taste of vine-ripened grapes in the summertime causes my mouth to water, it also makes my skin rejoice, for I know I can always set a few grapes aside as a gentle alpha-hydroxy treatment. The variety of delightful aromatic beauty treatments you can make with fresh fruits and vegetables is a surefire way to encourage you to find the time to pamper yourself, and to promote healthy eating habits.

Before getting started, note that each piece of fruit or vegetable has a different texture; for example, while one bunch of grapes is quite juicy, another is dry. This natural variety serves as fair warning that you may need to add a bit more or less of an ingredient than is called for in a particular recipe — always have a little extra on hand. This measure of slight unpredictability is part of the joy of making Aromatic Beauty Food; no two recipes are exactly alike, and you can alter each one to create your own individualized treats. (Refer to the following box for

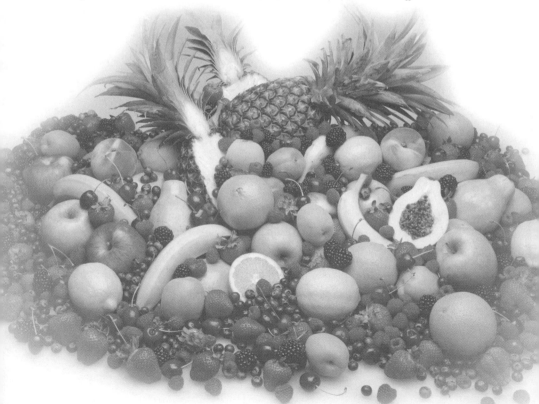

general information on varying recipes to account for the natural differences present in fresh foods.)

As you become more adept at making up your own recipes, you will be perfecting your instincts to mix and match these ingredients to create just the right texture for any product. Remember to always use fresh ingredients, and try to purchase foods that have been grown organically; you don't want to slather pesticides or growth hormones on your skin. Most of all, enjoy!

Aromatic Beauty Food Textures and Types

To make Aromatic Beauty Food, remember that the texture of a food product is what makes it suitable or unsuitable for one purpose or another. Refer to this information when you want to alter the recipes or create your own dreamy goodies.

~ **For finished products that are too runny,** add clay, ground or whole oats, ground almonds, cornmeal, flour, or fresh bread crumbs.

~ **For finished products with ingredients that refuse to cling together,** add banana, egg yolk, honey, room-temperature sour cream, yogurt, softened cream cheese, or softened butter.

~ **For finished products that are too dry and don't spread easily,** add hydrosol, distilled water, vegetable and/or fruit juice, whole or skim milk, melted ice cream, aloe vera gel, whipping cream, or sour cream.

~ **To make exfoliating products,** add amaranth, cornmeal, ground oats or almonds, wheat germ, semolina, dried coconut flakes, poppy seeds, sugar, cooked rice, or tapioca

~ **To help balance the pH of the skin,** add 1 teaspoon of apple cider vinegar to any cup of Aromatic Beauty Food.

Sara Phillips, Handmade Natural Soaps
Wells-next-the-Sea, Norfolk, England

Sara's expedition into the world of handmade toiletries began with one of the true pioneers of the industry, Barbara Bobo of Woodspirits Soaps. After seeing some of Barbara's soaps at a London exhibition, Sara was intrigued with the idea that she could make her own. But finding a soap-making book was no easy task for Sara. She had to travel 50 miles from home to request a book from a library, and waited more than three weeks for its arrival. It was nearly two months before she could finally try her hand at soap-making in her kitchen.

After a few disastrous attempts, Sara's perseverance paid off. She is now a self-described obsessive soapmaker. According to Sara, "Whenever I tell people I make soap, they say, 'Why, when you can buy it at the shops?' I just sigh quietly and start my spiel about the superiority of handmade soap!" Sara loves what her handmade soap does for her skin, and she's encouraged to see that a growing base of customers feel the same way. Her best-selling bar — which is also my favorite — is Cedar & Lemon, a blend of lemongrass, Litsea cubeba, and cedarwood.

When Sara creates the perfect bar of soap or tube of lip balm, she is absolutely thrilled. Her favorite essential oils are juniper needle, West Indian bay, frankincense, lime, lemon, and tea tree, and she plays around with them as often as she can, which is not often enough considering she is also a wife, mother of two small children, and the owner of a thriving graphic-design business!

What Are Alpha-Hydroxy Acids?

Alpha-hydroxy acids (AHAs) occur naturally in several foods and include citric acid (from citrus fruits), malic acid (from apples), tartaric acid (from grapes), lactic acid (from milk), and glycolic acid (from sugarcane). When applied to the skin, fruit acids supplement the skin's natural exfoliation process by loosening and sloughing away the outer layer of dead skin cells, revealing the newer, smoother cells underneath. This process rejuvenates the skin by improving circulation and stimulating new cell growth, resulting in a fresher, healthier complexion and reduced pore size.

Synthesized AHAs are used in over-the-counter cosmetics, and the FDA has issued guidelines suggesting that manufacturers refrain from incorporating concentrations of those synthesized AHAs in excess of 10 percent. Enjoy the benefits of fresh, natural alpha-hydroxy acids from grapes and apples in Face Food Fruit & Flowers (see page 140).

∼

Ah, you flavour everything, you are the vanille of society.

— Sydney Smith, *Lady Holland's Memoir*

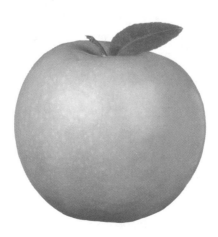

Face and Body Cleansers

These recipes were created to provide gentle alpha-hydroxy treatments and softly textured scrubs. Although most make enough product for one face and neck application, you can multiply the ingredients to make enough for your entire body.

Note: Be very careful using scrub-type products on broken or acne-scarred skin. Doing so could spread bacteria on the face, which could encourage further breakouts or leave scars. Either cleanse very gently or avoid these areas. If you have sensitive or sunburned skin, you should avoid scrubs.

HONEY GLEAM

This simple cleanser soothes and moisturizes normal to oily skin types. Use Honey Gleam as a quick, effective cleanser in the morning when you are in a hurry.

makes 1 application

1 egg white
2 tablespoons honey
1 teaspoon cornflower hydrosol
1 teaspoon whole milk or whipping cream

1. Whisk the egg white with a wire whisk or fork until slightly frothy. Add honey and stir well to incorporate.
2. Add cornflower hydrosol and milk or cream and stir well. If mixture seems a bit thick, add more hydrosol or milk. You don't want the mixture to be too thick, or you'll have to drag it across your skin.
3. To use, gently massage over face and neck skin, being careful not to pull at your skin. Rinse well, and follow with toner and moisturizer.

KIWI–ORANGE BLOSSOM PUREE

I love this facial cleanser for summer mornings when my oily skin calls for light cleansing. Of course, the best part about it is the taste, which, when combined with the light green color and visible flecks of kiwi seeds, makes an aesthetically pleasing fruit dip for a summertime party. Caution: Do not include the essential oils if you'll be snacking on this product.

makes 1 application

1 kiwi fruit
2 heaping tablespoons sour cream
1 tablespoon whole milk
1 tablespoon honey
1 heaping teaspoon finely ground almonds
1 drop orange essential oil
1 drop palmarosa essential oil

1. Puree about three quarters of the kiwi in a food processor until runny. Set aside the rest of the kiwi.
2. While processor is running, add sour cream, milk, honey, and almonds, and blend until thick and creamy, about 30 seconds.
3. Dip reserved kiwi piece into mixture, and eat!
4. Add essential oils last, then stir.
5. To use, massage gently over neck, face, and upper body to clean. Rinse well, and follow with toner and moisturizer.

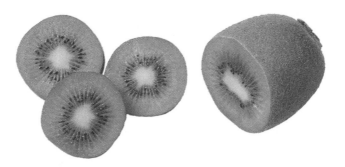

Nitty Gritty Grains

This lightly fragrant blend of gentle ingredients can be used to cleanse skin and gently stimulate circulation and exfoliation. In its dry form, it makes a great yogurt topping. Other ingredients you can use to customize Nitty Gritty Grains include fresh cucumber juice (for sensitive skin), sour cream (for oily and clogged skin), and honey and whipping cream (for dry skin).

makes approximately 10 applications, depending on if you add custom ingredients, and how much you use at one time

¼ cup oats, cut and sifted (not too finely ground)
¼ cup finely ground almonds
2 tablespoons finely ground cashews
2 tablespoons dried lavender buds
1 tablespoon amaranth or poppy seeds

1. Combine all ingredients, stirring well. Store in an airtight container until ready to use.
2. To use, scoop Nitty Gritty Grains into your palm and add enough of your favorite hydrosol or distilled water to make a gritty but moist, milky, pastelike substance. Massage over face and neck (avoiding eye area and broken skin) to cleanse and exfoliate. Rinse with warm water. Pat excess moisture from skin, and follow with toner and moisturizer.

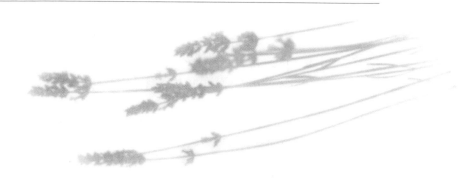

CUCUMBER WASH

Cucumber Wash, with a nice light lather provided by the soapwort, is very soothing and has light exfoliating properties.

makes 1 application

1 ounce dried soapwort root
1 tablespoon kaolin or other cosmetic
   clay of choice
1 tablespoon finely ground oats
½ medium-size cucumber, peeled
1 tablespoon sour cream
1 tablespoon soapwort root water
1 tablespoon spent soapwort root
1 teaspoon honey

1. Place about an ounce of dried soapwort root in a saucepan of cold water. Bring the water to a boil over low heat. Cover and simmer for about ½ hour.
2. Remove the pan from the heat and allow to cool, covered. Strain the liquid and reserve the root.
3. Mix together dry ingredients (kaolin and oats) in a bowl and set aside.
4. Pulverize the cucumber in a food processor or blender. Transfer to a second mixing bowl.
5. To the cucumber, add sour cream, soapwort root water, spent soapwort root, and honey. Stir well to mix and break up the sour cream.
6. Add dry ingredients and stir well to combine. Allow the mixture to stand for about 30 minutes, to thicken slightly before using.
7. To use, wet face and neck and wash with Cucumber Wash, using gentle, rounded strokes. Rinse with warm water, then repeat. Follow with toner and moisturizer.

BREAD OF LIFE
LAVENDER CLEANSER

*This mixture is refreshing, especially if left on the face
for a few minutes after applying. The gluten in the bread
produces a soft, pasty texture that is easily spread across
the skin to cleanse and lightly exfoliate. I sometimes use this recipe
in the morning to cleanse my entire body. Use Bread of Life
Lavender Cleanser immediately, as even overnight refrigeration
can result in an unpleasant, sour aroma.*

makes 1 whole-body application

> 2 ounces fresh whole-wheat or white bread, cut
> into small pieces
> ½ ounce crushed oats
> 1 teaspoon dried lavender buds
> 2 ounces lavender hydrosol
> 1 ounce aloe vera gel
> 1 teaspoon whipping cream
> 1 teaspoon honey
> 3 drops lavender essential oil
> 1 drop neroli essential oil

1. Place bread, oats, and lavender buds in mixing bowl and toss to combine.
2. Stir together all other ingredients, in a separate bowl, adding essentials oil last.
3. Add bread mixture to liquid ingredients and stir well to combine. If mixture is a bit runny, add a few more cubes of bread or some additional crushed oats to absorb some of the moisture. It should be the consistency of paste.
4. To use, scoop the mixture with your fingers, and apply to moistened skin with gently sweeping motions to cleanse.

Strawberry Morning
Face Frappé

*Use leftover Strawberry Morning Face Frappé
on your hands, or give it to a friend. The sweet smell
of strawberries and cream will brighten her day!*

makes approximately 2 applications

6 medium-size fresh strawberries, tops removed
1 small egg
1 tablespoon honey
⅛ lemon wedge, peeled and seeded
1 tablespoon wheat germ
1 tablespoon whipping cream
2 tablespoons lavender buds
1 tablespoon oats, finely ground
1 teaspoon kaolin
2 drops Tone Thyme (or other Aromatic Alchemy blend of choice; see pages 10–13)

1. Blend together 3 strawberries, the egg, honey, lemon, wheat germ, and whipping cream in a food processor for 1 minute while you eat one of the other strawberries. (Strawberries are wonderful natural "toothbrushes.")
2. Pour mixture into a bowl or cup. Add lavender, oats, kaolin, and Tone Thyme and stir to incorporate.
3. Eat another strawberry.
4. To use, apply this mixture to face upon rising, using gentle sweeping motions to cleanse. Rinse well, then reapply. Rinse again and pat face lightly dry. Follow with a few spritzes of the hydrosol of your choice, and apply a moisturizer.
5. Eat the last strawberry.

Kimberly Chance, Treasures from the Garden
Arlington, Texas

After earning a master's degree in social work and spending several years working with chronically ill patients, Kim discovered essential oils and their many uses. Ironically, it was Kim's patients who began telling her about the healing powers of the oils, and Kim was all too eager to listen.

The first product Kim made with essential oils was bath salts. Since then, she has graduated to making bath sizzles and soaks as well as lip balms. She first made these goodies for herself, but after giving samples to coworkers, Kim soon found herself receiving orders and Treasures from the Garden was born. Says Kim, "When I focus completely on what I'm doing, forgetting about trouble at work and elsewhere, it is really fun and rewarding to watch these little treats come together."

Kim has found that essential oils are a wonderful way to complement her clients' traditional medical treatments, and she is always careful to consult with the medical staff to ensure that none of the aromatics she suggests will conflict with any of her clients' medications or treatments. "It's fun to educate the physicians about essential oils, and I find myself encouraging them to educate themselves about aromatherapy in order to answer their patients' questions," she reports.

My favorite Treasures from the Garden product is Tropical Kiss Body Cream.

SUMMER MANGO COMPOTE

This simple compote will cleanse and refresh,
especially on a hot summer afternoon.

makes 1 application

½ small mango (about 2 ounces), flesh only
1 tablespoon honey
1 tablespoon whipping cream
2 tablespoons spent soapwort root (see page 134)

1. Blend mango flesh in food processor for 1 minute.
2. With processor running, add honey and whipping cream.
3. Add soapwort root last, and blend well. If your mango is extra juicy, you may wish to add some finely ground oats to absorb the excess juice.
4. To use, cup the mixture in your palms and apply to damp face and neck with gentle strokes. I like to refrigerate Summer Mango Compote for 1 hour before using it because the coolness is very refreshing.

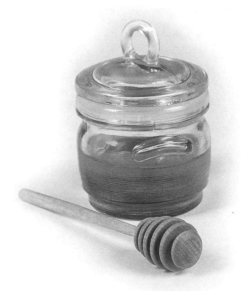

Tips for Enjoying Aromatic Beauty Food

To maximize enjoyment of your fresh creations, be sure to do the following:

- Pull as much of your hair as possible away from your face, or else you'll be combing food particles out of it for several minutes.
- Clean up quickly and thoroughly behind Aromatic Beauty Food — tiny food particles splash during use onto your carpet, the walls, behind the sink, and onto tiles.
- Use a drain strainer in the sink and bathtub to catch Aromatic Beauty Food particles that could cause clogs.
- Be careful when using Aromatic Beauty Food that contains oil-type ingredients, as the tub and shower area can become very slippery. You may feel more comfortable applying treatments while standing outside the tub or shower on a large plastic bag. Clean the shower and bathtub well following a treatment to make sure they do not remain slippery.
- Store Aromatic Beauty Food containing fresh cream, milk, and other perishables in the refrigerator, and use within a few days. Mixtures containing only dry ingredients (such as grains, oats, and powdered milk) can be stored indefinitely in airtight containers away from heat and light.

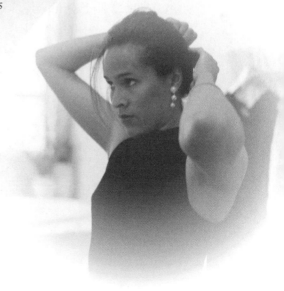

FACE FOOD FRUIT & FLOWERS

*This blend of goodies employs fresh alpha- and beta-hydroxy acids
to cleanse and tone the skin. Bonus: A clayless, essential-oil-less
version of this recipe makes a wonderful dip for fruit!*

makes 1 full-body application

½ cup whole rolled oats
½ cup cashews, finely ground
¼ cup amaranth
¼ cup freshly juiced apple juice
¼ cup freshly juiced grape juice
¼ cup freshly juiced pineapple juice
2 tablespoons whipping cream
At least 1 chunk of your favorite fresh fruit
Enough kaolin or other clay to thicken the mixture
   to a smooth paste
2 drops Face Flowers (see page 10)

1. Combine oats, cashew meal, and amaranth in a bowl. Add
   fresh juices and whipping cream and stir well to combine.
2. Dip your fresh fruit chunks, and enjoy a refreshing treat.
3. Add kaolin to remaining mixture and stir until a smooth paste
   forms. Incorporate essential oil.
4. To use, massage over face in gentle, circular motions. Rinse
   well and gently pat dry.

ESTHER'S BEAUTY PUDDING

Named for the biblical queen who, after being pampered and bathed in fragrant oils for two years, was sent by God to save her people from destruction, Esther's Beauty Pudding is a really satisfying treat. I like to use this as a morning cleanser on days when my skin feels especially dry.

makes approximately 2 generous applications

1 cup whipping cream
¼ cup whole rolled oats
1 teaspoon sandalwood hydrosol
1 teaspoon rose hydrosol
1 drop frankincense essential oil
1 drop myrrh essential oil, *or* 3 drops
    Tender Warrior (see page 11)

1. Heat whipping cream over a very low flame until warm, but not hot to the touch. (Test it by removing a spoonful and touching it lightly with your fingertips.) Do not scald the whipping cream.
2. Add oats, and stir until mixture becomes a pudding. Remove from heat.
3. Add hydrosols and essential oils and stir well to incorporate.
4. To use, gently apply warm mixture to face, neck, and decolletage area, using upward, sweeping motions to cleanse the face. If desired, leave some of the mixture on your skin and rest for 15 minutes. Breathe deeply to enjoy the aromatics, and relax. Rinse, then follow with toner and moisturizer. I like to use Melissa-Rose Second Skin Elixir (see page 114) after this cleanser. Refrigerate any leftovers for up to a few days.

Body Scrubs

Body scrubs are made with textured ingredients that help slough away dead skin. They feel great, and make your skin soft and silky.

FEET TENDERIZER

If you've been spending an extra $5 or $10 at the spa for a paraffin wax to soften and soothe extremely rough feet, get ready to save some money. Store spent coffee grounds in the refrigerator to make this treatment when you're ready. Do not use this scrub on sensitive or damaged skin.

makes 1 application for each foot

3 tablespoons finely ground spent coffee grounds
1 teaspoon cornmeal
1 teaspoon extra-virgin olive oil
1 tablespoon whipping cream
1 tablespoon whole-wheat, rice, or white flour
2 drops lavender essential oil
2 drops tea tree essential oil

1. Measure coffee grounds and cornmeal into a small bowl, and stir in the olive oil.
2. Add whipping cream and flour and stir well to make a thin paste.
3. Add essential oil and stir to incorporate.
4. To use, hold foot over sink or tub and scoop up about a quarter of the mixture. Scrub onto skin, being careful to include the soles, balls of feet and heels, and your entire hand. Rinse each extremity as you go. Don't scrub too hard or your skin may become irritated. Rinse feet well and gently pat skin dry with a soft towel. Always follow this treatment with a rich, soothing moisturizer such as Ballerina Butter (page 102).

ROSEMARY'S APPLE CRISP BODY SCRUB

This mix of apple juice and "crunchies" forms a luxurious whole-body exfoliant that is moisturizing and soothing. "Age" the mixture in the refrigerator for at least 8 hours before using.

makes 1 application

5 tablespoons whipping cream

1 tablespoon honey

3 tablespoons freshly juiced apple juice

4 tablespoons tapioca pearls

2 tablespoons whole rolled oats, lightly crushed

1 cup Epsom salts or coarse sea salt

1 drop rose essential oil

1 drop neroli essential oil

2 drops palmarosa essential oil

2 drops lemon peel essential oil, or
 5 drops Balancing Act (see page 12)

1. Warm whipping cream in microwave for about 15 seconds. Remove from the microwave.
2. Add honey and apple juice, then stir to combine.
3. Add tapioca and oats, then stir.
4. Add salts and stir well.
5. Add essential oils and stir.
6. To use, stand naked in a dry bathtub and scoop some of the mixture in your palms. Beginning with your extremities, gently scrub your skin in circular motions, moving up your leg to your thigh, and from your hands to your shoulders. If you have a helper to scrub your back, all the better! This scrub is even gentle enough to smooth over your breasts (avoid the nipples) and lower neck area. Rinse off and pat dry with a towel.

GINGER CRUSH BODY POLISH

*This treatment will stimulate circulation, gently exfoliate skin,
and help rid the body of toxins. Store for up to four weeks in the
refrigerator, preferably in a glass container
with a tightly fitting screw-top lid.*

makes 1 application

1 cup Epsom salts or coarse sea salt
¼ cup dried lavender buds
¼ cup dried calendula petals
¼ cup kelp
¼ cup poppy seeds
¼ cup cornmeal
½ cup sweet almond oil
⅛ cup fresh ginger juice
¼ cup freshly juiced orange juice
10 drops orange essential oil (note citrus oil
and sun exposure caution, page 25)
8 drops lavender essential oil
1 drop Roman chamomile essential oil

1. Combine salts, lavender, calendula, kelp, poppy seeds, and cornmeal and set aside.
2. Combine sweet almond oil, juices, and essential oils in a separate container. Add oils to salt mixture and stir well.
3. To use, stand naked in a dry bathtub, and, beginning with your extremities, massage the treatment by the handful into your skin. If some slips through your fingers, just pick it up and keep scrubbing. I like to use this in a steamy bathroom. Avoid massaging into delicate areas such as face and genitals. After use, rinse and gently towel try.

Face and Body Masks

Masks can be made with clay, which draws toxins from the skin, or with pectin, which soothes and smoothes. These recipes will get you started on creating your own masks using the fresh foods that are best for your skin type.

TOTALLY COOL FACE MASK

This all-purpose skin mask has thousands of variations.
It is made with pectin, a natural thickening agent. To make the
base, combine the first three ingredients as shown below, making
substitutions if you desire. For example, substitute herbal tea
or hydrosol, or a combination of the two, for the hot water.
To select ingredients for your skin type, refer to page 61
for hydrosols and pages 51–52 for herbs.

makes 1 application

1 ounce (28 g) vegetable glycerin
1 ounce hot water (or herbal infusion
  and/or hydrosol)
1 ounce pectin
1 drop Aromatic Alchemy blend of choice
  (see pages 10–13) (optional)

1. Dissolve the glycerin in water by stirring well. Using an electric mixer on low speed, slowly add the pectin to the water-glycerin mixture. Stir until mixture begins to thicken.
2. Allow to sit for about ½ hour so a gel can form. Add Aromatic Alchemy blend, if desired.
3. To use, apply to clean face and neck, avoiding eye and mouth areas. Rest for 10 minutes. Rinse with warm water, and follow with toner and moisturizer.

FRUIT FOUNDATIONS

Fruit Foundations, a luscious mélange of fruits, whipping cream, and aromatic oils, not only is a soothing facial mask to remove excess oil from the surface of the skin but also makes a tasty addition to your snack tray.

makes 1 application

6 ounces (170 g) fresh fruit chunks peeled (pineapples, kiwis, seedless grapes, and assorted melons are good choices; grapes need not be peeled but should be rinsed)
1 ounce (28 g) whipping cream
1 teaspoon honey
½ ounce (14 g) kaolin
1 drop rose essential oil
1 drop sandalwood essential oil

1. Place mixed fruits in food processor or blender, and blend until juicy but not liquefied, about 20 seconds.
2. Add whipping cream and honey, and blend another 15 seconds.
3. Separate out 2 ounces (about 4 heaping tablespoons) of the fruit-cream-honey mixture, add the clay and essential oils to it, and stir to make a paste. (Set aside the rest of the mixture, without the clay and oil, and use it as a dip or ice cream topping. I like to add a handful of crushed almonds or cashews, too . . . yum!)
4. To use, apply to clean face and neck, avoiding eye and mouth areas. Rest for 10 minutes. Rinse with warm water, and follow with toner and moisturizer.

BREAKFAST SPREAD

A most refreshing and creamy, skin-soothing treat. Spread leftovers
on your toasted sesame seed bagel!

makes 1 application

½ small tangerine, peeled and seeded,
   or 2 drops Tender Warrior (see page 11)
2 ounces softened cream cheese

1. Mash the tangerine flesh with the back of a fork. Add tangerine flesh to softened cream cheese and stir well to incorporate.
   Reserve 1 teaspoon of Breakfast Spread, and enjoy it with your
   English muffin and tea.
2. To use, apply to clean face and neck, avoiding eye and mouth
   areas. Rest for 10 minutes. Rinse with warm water, and follow
   with toner and moisturizer.

STRAWBERRY-ROSE
FACIAL CUSTARD

This recipe is fresh and cooling and is especially good for oily skin.

makes 1 application

6 strawberries (tops removed), mashed
2 tablespoons sour cream
1 tablespoon flour
1 teaspoon honey
1 drop rose essential oil, or 1 drop
   Balancing Act (see page 12)

1. Stir ingredients into a smooth paste.
2. Apply evenly to face and neck. Relax for 20 minutes. Rinse
   with warm water, and follow with toner and moisturizer.

CUCUMBER-AVOCADO
CLAY MASK

*This recipe is courtesy of Rosalind Sledd, who created it at last
year's Aromatic Beauty Workshop in Chicago. Rosalind chose not
to add essential oils, preferring this combination of goodies
"in the buff." It smelled just like a fresh vegetable salad,
and I felt healthier simply because I sniffed it!*

makes 1 application

¼ cup cucumber, peeled and chopped
¼ cup avocado flesh
1 teaspoon sour cream
1 teaspoon plain yogurt
3 tablespoons coarsely ground rolled oats
4 teaspoons pink clay or other clay of choice
1 tablespoon lime juice
1 teaspoon honey
1 teaspoon dried lavender buds

1. Puree the cucumber and avocado flesh in food processor until smooth.
2. Add each of the other ingredients, one at a time in the order shown, and process briefly after each addition.
3. To use, apply to clean face and neck, avoiding eye and mouth areas. Rest for 10 minutes. Rinse with warm water and follow with toner and moisturizer.

Cereal Thriller Oatmeal Mask

For dry skin, add 2 drops of Face Flowers Aromatic Alchemy blend (see page 10) to ¼ cup cooked oatmeal. Apply a layer to clean face and neck skin, and rest for 10 minutes. Rinse well, and follow with moisturizer.

HONEY-APRICOT BODY BRÛLÉE

I like to apply this soothing mask of goodies before a special occasion. For a treat, warm the finished mixture in the microwave for about 15 seconds before adding aromatic oils. This is a very soothing whole-body mask, and the apricot blends well with Roman chamomile essential oil to lightly perfume the skin.

makes 1 application

> 1 apricot, peeled and seeded
> 1 tablespoon honey
> ¼ cup whipping cream
> 1 tablespoon finely ground rolled oats
> 1 tablespoon finely ground almonds
> 1 teaspoon kaolin
> 2 drops Roman chamomile essential oil, or
>   2 drops Drench (see page 13)

1. Blend apricot in food processor until smooth. While doing this, warm the honey and whipping cream in the microwave on high setting for about 15 seconds (you want the mixture to be warm and pourable, but not hot). Add the honey-cream mixture to the apricot and blend.
2. Add the oats, almonds, and kaolin, and process until smooth. You can warm the mixture for about 15 seconds in the microwave on high setting at this point, if desired.
3. Stir in essential oil.
4. To use, apply to clean face and neck, avoiding eye and mouth areas. Rest for 10 minutes. Rinse with warm water, and follow with toner and moisturizer.

THE BACK PACK

*This mask, which is best for normal to oily skin,
gently draws impurities and toxins from the surface of
hard-to-reach and often neglected back skin. For best
results, a friend can apply this for you.*

makes 1 application

3 tablespoons witch hazel hydrosol
1 teaspoon vegetable glycerin
4 tablespoons green clay or other very
drawing clay
1 drop ylang ylang essential oil
2 drops lemon essential oil
(note citrus oil caution, page 25)
2 drops geranium essential oil, or
3 drops Tone Thyme (see page 12)

1. Combine witch hazel hydrosol and vegetable glycerin and stir until glycerin dissolves.
2. Add liquid mixture to clay and stir well to form a creamy paste. Add aromatic oils and stir well.
3. To use, have another person apply a thin to medium layer of The Back Pack to your entire clean back area while you lie on your stomach. Relax for 10 minutes until the mask dries. Rinse well, and follow with a spritz of the hydrosol of your choice and a light moisturizer.

BANANA MOON

There's nothing like giving yourself a facial using ingredients that are likely to be in your kitchen year-round. Except for the essential oils in this recipe, you surely have all the ingredients in your cupboard, or can easily obtain them in a flash! This will leave any type of skin feeling refreshed and pampered.

makes 1 application

1 banana, just ripe
1 tablespoon honey
1 egg yolk
1 teaspoon wheat germ oil
1 tablespoon finely powdered oats
1 teaspoon lemon juice (optional,
    if mask will not be used immediately)
1 drop each rose and melissa essential oil,
    or 2 drops Balancing Act (see page 12)

1. Peel and mash banana. Add honey, egg yolk, wheat germ oil, oats, and lemon juice, if used, and mash further to form a smooth, creamy paste.
2. If mask is too thick, add a bit of distilled water or hydrosol of choice, and stir well until smooth.
3. Add essential oils last, and stir to mix well.
4. To use, apply to clean face and neck, avoiding eye and mouth areas. Rest for 10 minutes, or longer if your skin is very dry. Rinse with warm water, and follow with toner and moisturizer. Use application within a few hours of making.

THE PRINCESS PACK

A mask and exfoliant in one, The Princess Pack is a royal treatment that will leave your skin feeling soft and supple.

makes 1 application

1 egg yolk
1 tablespoon milk or whipping cream
1 teaspoon honey
2 tablespoons oats, finely ground
1 tablespoon kaolin or other clay
1 drop each lavender and sandalwood essential oil, or 2 drops Face Flowers (see page 10)

1. Whisk egg yolk with wire whisk or fork. Add milk or cream and honey, then whisk again.
2. Add oats and kaolin, and stir well to form a smooth mixture. Allow mixture to stand a few minutes to firm up a bit.
3. To use, apply to clean face and neck, avoiding eye and mouth areas. Rest for 10 minutes, or longer if your skin is very dry. Rinse with warm water, and follow with toner and moisturizer.

Beauty and the Bees

In antiquity, honey was regarded as a gift from the heavens, and it was widely believed that it simply rained from the sky and was collected by bees. Pliny the Elder called honey "saliva from the stars," and evidence of medicinal and cosmetic uses of honey has been found in Egyptian tombs, where the first recorded beehives are artfully detailed. Everyone from God to Winnie-the-Pooh touts the virtues of honey. In my opinion, no Aromatic Beauty Food routine is complete without it.

PASSION FRUIT POTION

This mask contains passion fruit, one of my favorite summertime treats. The slippery, glutinous substance that covers the passion-fruit seeds make the fruit especially suitable for facial masks. Passion Fruit Potion is designed for drier skin types. Most upscale grocery stores carry passion fruit in the summer.

makes 1 application

Inner seeds and pulp from 1 passion fruit
  (see directions below)
1 teaspoon honey
½ teaspoon elderflower hydrosol
1 tablespoon kaolin
1 drop each sandalwood and jasmine essential
  oil, or 2 drops Mercy (see page 11)

1. To remove the seeds and flesh from the passion fruit, lop off one end of the fruit, cutting through to the white inner rind. Scoop out the flesh and seeds.
2. Place the flesh and seeds in a small bowl, then add honey and hydrosol. Stir to incorporate.
3. Add the kaolin, and stir again until smooth.
4. Add aromatic oils last, and stir once again.
5. To use, apply to clean face and neck, avoiding eye and mouth areas. Rest for 10 minutes. Rinse with warm water, and follow with toner and moisturizer.

TOMATO TUNE-UP
FACIAL TONER

This pretty pink potion will tone and smooth oily skin.
This recipe does not keep well in the refrigerator,
so divide it in half and share it with a friend.

makes 2 applications

1 small, ripe tomato
⅛ peeled lemon, pulp and pith removed
1 tablespoon sour cream
1 egg white
1 teaspoon honey
½ teaspoon xanthan gum
1 drop each lemon and cypress essential oil,
    or 2 drops Tone Thyme (see page 12;
    these oils are optional)

1. Process tomato in food processor until liquid, about 2 minutes.
2. Add lemon, sour cream, egg white, and honey, and process until smooth, about 1 minute. The tomato seeds and skin pieces will be visible.
3. Add xanthan gum and process 1 more minute. The xanthan gum will thicken the mixture.
4. Stir in essential oil, if using.
5. To use, stir vigorously to mix. Pat over clean face and neck area. Do not rub in. After 5 to 7 minutes, you will feel your pores begin to tighten. After a few more minutes, rinse well with warm water. Pat excess water from face and apply some moisturizer.

Body Butters and Moisturizers

These rich, buttery treats will provide a whole new way to view food. Until you've tried smoothing avocado pulp or peanut butter onto dry skin, you just haven't lived as a cosmeti-cook!

NEWLYWED BUTTER

Not only is this an exquisite body treat for yourself, but also it tastes fantastic, which makes it an especially wonderful fresh gift to pack for the bride and groom.

makes 1 application

> 2 heaping tablespoons crunchy peanut butter
> 1 tablespoon white sugar
> 2 teaspoons honey
> 1 teaspoon virgin coconut oil
> 1 tablespoon distilled water

1. In a bowl, mix all ingredients well to combine. If the mixture is not smooth (except for the peanut pieces), add more water until a smooth consistency is obtained.
2. To use, stand naked in the tub, scoop the mixture into your palms, and massage over your skin's surface, starting with extremities and working toward the center of the body. The peanuts and sugar provide gentle exfoliation, while the rest of the ingredients soothe and nourish. Shower, using a gentle handmade cleanser to remove the butter. Pat skin lightly dry as usual, and follow with moisturizer if desired.

BETTER BODY BUTTER

This is far and away the most popular recipe at Aromatic Beauty Workshops, and it works better than any commercial body butter I have ever used. Whether in winter or summer, people love smoothing this delicious goody all over their hands and arms. I usually save this recipe for last in the workshops because it causes such a stir.

makes 1 application

1 ripe banana
Flesh of 1 ripe avocado
1 stick softened sweet butter
¼ cup whipping cream
1 drop rose essential oil, or
1 drop Saving Face (see page 13)

1. Blend the ingredients one at a time in a food processor until smooth. If necessary, add more whipping cream to make the mixture smooth and silky. If you don't have a food processor, you can use a food masher or your hands, but you will not attain the smooth texture that makes this product so sensual.

2. To use, steam the bathroom to open your pores and prepare your skin for the treatment. Place an old blanket on the bathroom floor, and put two large plastic trash bags together, end to end, on top of the blanket. Massage Better Body Butter over the entire body, avoiding eye area and any open wounds. You can also spread this luscious concoction over your face, especially if you have dry skin.

3. Lie down on the trash bags, and wrap yourself in them and the blanket, being careful not to get any of the mixture on carpeting. Close your eyes and dream for about 15 minutes. Rinse off in the shower, using a soft cloth or bath puff and a handmade soap with a luxurious lather. Feel beautiful!

Resources

Raw Materials, Packaging & Body-Care Products

Acme Vial & Glass Company
800-394-2745
www.acmevial.com

Acqua Vita
866-405-8855
www.acqua-vita.com
Hydrosols

Alban Muller International
305-994-7558
www.albanmuller.com
Herbal extracts, oils, and butters

Arista Industries
800-255-6457
www.aristaindustries.com
Oils and butters

Aromatherapy Place
800-327-2025
www.auroma.com
Aromatics, raw materials, books, and classes

Camden-Grey Essential Oils
888-207-9724
www.camdengrey.com

Columbus Foods Company
800-322-6457
www.columbusfoods.com
Oils

E. D. Luce Prescription Packaging
562-802-0515
www.essentialsupplies.com
Wholesale bottles, vials, jars, and apothecary supplies

Enfleurage
888-387-0300
www.enfleurage.com
Aromatics and books

Essence of Life
505-758-7941
www.sacredoilsofkrishna.com
Indian aromatics and classes

Essential Oil Company
800-729-5912
www.essentialoil.com
Aromatics and florasols

From Nature With Love
800-520-2060
www.fromnaturewithlove.com
Raw materials

Gentle Emu Oil Products
877-436-8537
www.gentleridge.com
Emu oil and handmade soap

Jean's Greens
518-479-0471
www.jeansgreens.com
Herbs and herbal extracts

Lebermuth Company
800-648-1123
www.lebermuth.com
Aromatics, accessories, and herbs

Majestic Mountain Sage
801-227-0837
www.the-sage.com
Raw materials

Milky Way Molds
503-482-5056
www.milkywaymolds.com

Nature's Gift
615-612-4270
www.naturesgift.com
Aromatics and books

Nectarine
800-966-3457
www.nectarine.biz
Aromatics and packaging

Oils of Aloha
800-367-6010
www.oilsofaloha.com
Kukui and Macadamia oils

Original Swiss Aromatics
415-459-3998
www.originalswissaromatics.com
Aromatics

Prima Fleur
415-455-0957
www.primafleur.com
Aromatics

Purcell Natural Jojoba
800-676-1501
www.purcelljojoba.com
Jojoba oil

Rainbow Meadow
800-207-4047
www.rainbowmeadow.com
Aromatics and raw materials

Samara Bontane
800-782-4532
www.wingedseed.com
Essential oils and accessories

Sensory Essence
847-526-3645
www.organicbulgarianrose.com
Bulgarian aromatics

SKS Bottle and Packaging
518-880-6980, ext. 1
www.sks-bottle.com

Starwest Botanicals
800-800-4372
www.starwest-botanicals.com
Bulk herbs, essential oils, and
herbal extracts

Summers Past Farms
619-390-1523
www.summerspastfarms.com
Herbs, aromatics, and classes

Sun Feather Natural Soap Co.
315-265-3648
www.sunsoap.com
Aromatics, base oils and fats,
books, and videos

Sunburst Bottle Company
916-929-4500
www.sunburstbottle.com

A Woman of Uncommon Scents
800-377-3685
www.awomanofuncommonscents.com
Aromatics

Woodspirits Ltd.
937-663-4327
www.woodspirits.com
Handmade soap

Contact Information for Profiled
Toiletries Makers

Andrea Fowler
Country Herbals by Andrea
570-996-0910
www.countryherbals.com

Connie Henrie
No longer in business

Ginny Lee
**Ginny Lee Natural Face & Body
Products**
No longer in business

Jan Berger
Body Way
No longer in business

Kimberly Chance
Treasures from the Garden
No longer in business

Leslie Plant
Leslie's Garden Handcrafted Soap
301-779-8562
www.lesliesgarden.com

Marti Cook
Cook's Cottage Farm
No longer in business

Melody Upham
Rainbow Meadow, Inc.
800-207-4047
www.rainbowmeadow.com

Pat Silver
No longer in business

Sara Phillips
The Natural Soap Company
Formerly Handmade Natural Soaps
+44-0-1-328-711-717
www.naturalsoap.co.uk

Vicki Bedell
Welstar
Formerly Essential Restoratives
800-893-6008
www.welstar.net

Index

Page numbers in *italics* indicate charts.

O/W and W/O emulsions, 75–76, 77
storing, 21, 37, 41, 48
types of, 3, 5
See also Aromatic oils; Essential oils; Health warnings: oils; Unscented oils
Oily skin, 12, 29, 31, 32, 41, 46, 57, 33
Olive oil (*Olea europaea*), 45–46

Palm stearic acid (*Elaeis guineensis*), 82
Patchouli (*Pogostemon cablin, P. heyeanus* syn. *patchouli*), 28
Patch test, 8, 46, 58
Peanut oil (*Arachis hypogaea*), 46
Petroleum jelly, 45
Phillips, Sara, 129
Photosensitivity, 25
Phytols/phytosols (now florasols), 18
Plantain (*Plantago major*), 51
Plant, Leslie, 53
Plant water. *See* Hydrosol/hydrolat
Popsicle sticks, 74
Psoriasis, 50

Queen of Flowers. *See* Rose oil

Rainbow Meadow, Inc., 43
Roman chamomile oil (*Chamaemelum nobile*), 23–24
Rooibos (*Aspalathus linearis*), 51
Rose hips (*Rosa rubiginosa*) seed CO₂ extract, 29
Rose hips seed oil (*Rosa rubiginosa, R. moschata, R. canina*), 46
Rosemary oil (*Rosmarinus officinalis*), 29
Rose oil/Queen of Flowers (*Rosa* x *damascena, R.* x

alba, R. x *centifolia*), 28

Safety guidelines. *See* Health warnings
Safflower oil (*Carthamus tinctorius*), 46
Sallow skin, 13, 24, 49
Sandalwood (*Santalum album*), 29–30
Scars, 29, 41, 116, 123
Sea buckthorn (*Hippophae rhamnoides*) berry CO₂ extract, 30
Second Skin Elixirs, 114–17
Sedatives, 30
Sensitive skin, 33, 57
Separation, of emulsions, 70
Sesame seed oil (*Sesamum indicum*), 46
Sexual desire, 34
Shea butter (*Butyrosperum parkii*), 45, 47
Shelf-life, 37, 40, 48, 90
Silver, Pat, 124
Skin irritations, 42, 51–52, 125
  burns, 23, 25, 41, 50, 51
  eczema, 50, 51, 125
  inflammations, 11, 23, 25, 31, 41, 46, 51, 52, 116
  insect bites, 23, 51
Smoking, 55
Soaps, 34, 40, 82
SPF (sun protection factor), 60
Spikenard oil (*Nardostachys jataamansi*), 30
Spent plant material, 15
Sprains, 41
Squalene (squalane), 47
Steam bath, facial, 65
Steam distillation, 15
St.-John's-wort (*Hypericum perforatum*), 51–52
Storing products, 21, 37, 41, 48, 74–75
Stress, 27, 28, 126
Sun, 25, 50, 60
Sunflower seed oil (*Helianthus annuus*), 47
Suppliers, 37, 157–60
Sweet almond oil (*Prunus*

dulcis), 47–48

Tamanu/foraha oil (*Calophyllum inophyllum*), 48
Teas, herb, 50
Tea tree oil (*Melaleuca alternifolia*), 31
Thickeners, 78–80, 82–85, 114
Thyme (*Thymus vulgaris*), 31
Toners, 24, 25, 60, 63–64
Tragacanth gum (*Astragalus* spp., *A. gummifer*), 83
Treasures from the Garden, 137
T-zone, 58

Unscented oils
  botanicals, 49–52
  list of, 38–42, 44–48
  origin of, 36–37
Upham, Melody, 43

Vascular conditions, 24
Vegetable emulsifying wax, 84
Vitamins A, C or E, 42, 46, 47, 48–49
Volatility rate, 6

Water botanicals, 49–50
Water phase, 85–86
Wax, 16–17, 78–79, 79–80, 84, 87
Weight conversions, 72
Wheat germ oil (*Triticum* spp.), 48
Witch hazel (*Hamamelis virginiana*), 52
W/O (water-in-oil) emulsions, 75–76, 77
Wrinkles. *See* Face care: mature skin

Xanthan gum, 84–85

Yarrow oil (*Achillea millefolium*), 31, 52
Ylang ylang oil (*Cananga odorata* var. *genuina*), 32

Other Storey Titles You Will Enjoy

The Aromatherapy Companion, by Victoria H. Edwards.
The most comprehensive aromatherapy guide, filled with profiles of
essential oils and recipes for beauty, health, and well-being.
288 pages. Paper. ISBN 978-1-58017-150-2.

The Essential Oils Book: Creating Personal Blends for Mind & Body,
by Colleen K. Dodt.
A rich resource on the many uses of aromatherapy and its applications
in everyday life.
160 pages. Paper. ISBN 978-0-88266-913-7.

The Herbal Home Remedy Book, by Joyce A. Wardwell.
A wealth of herbal healing wisdom, with advice on how to collect and
store herbs, make remedies, and stock a home herbal medicine chest.
176 pages. Paper. ISBN 978-1-58017-016-1.

**The Herbal Home Spa: Naturally Refreshing Wraps, Rubs, Lotions,
Masks, Oils, and Scrubs,** by Greta Breedlove.
A collection of easy-to-create personal care products that rival potions
found at exclusive spas and specialty shops.
208 pages. Paper. ISBN 978-1-58017-005-5.

Natural Foot Care, by Stephanie Tourles.
A comprehensive handbook natural, homemade herbal treatments,
massage techniques, and exercises for healthy feet.
192 pages. Paper. ISBN 978-1-58017-054-3.

Naturally Healthy Skin, by Stephanie Tourles.
A total reference about caring for all types of skin, with recipes,
techniques, and practical advice.
208 pages. Paper. ISBN 978-1-58017-130-4.

Organic Body Care Recipes, by Stephanie Tourles.
Homemade, herbal formulas for glowing skin, hair, and nails, plus
a vibrant self.
384 pages. Paper. ISBN 978-1-58017-676-7.

These and other books from Storey Publishing are available
wherever quality books are sold or by calling 1-800-441-5700.
Visit us at *www.storey.com*.